Stedman's

UROLOGY

WORDS

Williams & Wilkins

BALTIMORE • PHILADELPHIA • HONG KONG
LONDON • MUNICH • SYDNEY • TOKYO

A WAVERLY COMPANY

Series Editor: Elizabeth Randolph
Editor: Betsy Dearborn
Production Manager: Cordelia Slaughter
Cover Design: Carla Frank

Copyright © 1993
Williams & Wilkins
428 East Preston Street
Baltimore, Maryland 21202, USA

Printed in the United States of America

Library of Congress Cataloging-in-Publication Data
Stedman's urology words.
    p. cm.
    Developed from the database of Stedman's medical dictionary, 25th ed., and supplemented by terminology found in the current medical literature.
    Includes bibliographical references.
    ISBN 0-683-07960-3
    1. Urology—Terminology. I. Stedman, Thomas Lathrop, 1853–1938. Medical dictionary. II. Title: Urology words.
    [DNLM: 1. Urology—terminology. 2. Urologic Diseases—terminology. WJ 15 S799 1993]
RC871.S74 1993
616.6′003—dc20
DNLM/DLC
for Library of Congess   93-11350
                                             CIP

                             93 94 95 96 97
            1 2 3 4 5 6 7 8 9 10

Contents

Acknowledgments

An important part of our editorial process is the involvement of medical transcriptionists—as advisors, reviewers and/or editors. Betsy Dearborn did an excellent job once again of editing and proofing the manuscript and compiling the appendices. Other medical transcriptionist contributors to **Stedman's Urology Words** include: Sandy Kovacs, CMT; Averill Ring, CMT; Lenore Daniel; and Vicki Willms.

As with all our Stedman's word references, we have benefited from the words, suggestions and expertise of our many contacts in the medical transcriptionist community. Thanks to all our advisory board participants, reviewers and editors, and AAMT meeting attendees, and others who have written in with requests and comments—keep talking, and we'll keep listening.

Explanatory Notes

Stedman's Urology Words offers an authoritative assurance of quality and exactness to the wordsmiths of the health care professions—medical transcriptionists, medical editors and copy editors, medical records personnel, and the many other users and producers of medical documentation. It can be used to validate both the spelling and accuracy of terminology in urology. This compilation of over 12,000 entries, fully cross-indexed for quick access, was built from a base vocabulary of medical words, phrases, abbreviations and acronyms. The extensive A-Z list was developed from the database of **Stedman's Medical Dictionary, 25ed**. and supplemented by terminology found in the current medical literature.

Medical transcription is an art as well as a science. Both are needed to correctly interpret a physician's dictation, whose language is a product of education, training, and experience. This variety in medical language means that there are several acceptable ways to express certain terms, including jargon. **Stedman's Urology Words** provides variant spellings and phrasings for many terms. This, in addition to complete cross-indexing, makes **Stedman's Urology Words** a valuable resource for determining the validity of cardiology terms as they are encountered.

Stedman's Urology Words includes up-to-date terminology of the specialty, including genitourinary surgery, laparoscopic urology, endourology, urolithology and lithotripsy, renography, ultrasonography, male infertility, urogynecology and fluorourodynamics, and pediatric urology. The user will find listed thousands of diseases and syndromes, diagnostic and surgical procedures, tests, abbreviations, and eponymic terms. Drugs and equipment names related to urology are also included.

Alphabetical Organization

Alphabetization of entries is letter by letter as spelled, ignoring punctuation, spaces, prefixed numbers, Greek letters, or other characters. For example:

acid-fast staining methods
acid formaldehyde hematin
α-acid glycoprotein
acid hematin

In subentries, the abbreviated singular form or the spelled-out plural form of the noun main entry word is ignored in alphabetization.

Format and Style

All main entries are in **boldface** to speed up location of a sought-after entry, to enhance distinction between main entries and subentries, and to relieve the textual density of the pages.

Irregular plurals and variant spellings are shown on the same line as the singular or preferred form of the word. For example:

perineum, pl. **perinea**

caliceal, calyceal
  c. diverticulum
  c. extension
  c. fornix
  c. infundibulum

Possessive forms that occur in the medical literature are retained in this reference. To form the non-possessives advocated by the American Association for Medical Transcription and other groups, simply drop the apostrophe or apostrophe "s" from the end of the word. It should be noted that eponymic equipment and instrument names frequently appear in non-possessive form.

Cross-indexing

The word list is in an index-like main entry-subentry format that contains two combined alphabetical listings:

(1) A noun main entry-subentry organization typical of the A-Z section of medical dictionaries like **Stedman's**:

hernia
antevesical h.
direct inguinal h.
indirect inguinal h.
inguinal h.
inguinoscrotal h.

pyeloplasty
Anderson-Hynes pl
capsular flap p.
Culp p.
Culp spiral flap p.
disjoined p.

(2) An adjective main entry-subentry organization, which lists words and phrases as you hear them. The main entries are the adjectives or modifiers descriptors in a multi-word term. The subentries are the nouns around which the terms are constructed and to which the adjectives or descriptors pertain:

calcium
c. ATPase pump
c. carbonate
c. chloride
c. entry blocker
c. oxalate

voiding
v. cystogram
v. cystometrography
v. cystometry
v. cystourethrogram
v. diary

This format provides the user with more than one way to locate and identify a multi-word term. For example:

prosthesis
Flexi-Flate II penile p.

Flexi-Flate
F.-F. II penile
prosthesis

lesion
acetowhite l.

acetowhite
a. lesion

It also allows the user to see together all terms that contain a particular modifier as well as all types, kinds, or variations of a noun entity. For example:

bypass
aortorenal b.
b. graft
hepatorenal b.
iliorenal b.

kidney
k. allograft
artificial k.
Ask-Upmark k.
cadaver k.
k. carbuncle

Wherever possible, abbreviations are defined and cross-referenced throughout. For example:

KLH
keyhole limpet hemocyanin

hemocyanin
keyhole limpet h. (KLH)

keyhole
k. limpet hemocyanin (KLH)

References

Clayman RV and McDougall EM. Laparoscopic urology. St. Louis: Quality Medical Publishing; 1993.

Crawford ED and Das S, Current GU. Cancer surgery. Baltimore: Williams & Wilkins; 1990.

Hashmat AI and Das S. The penis. Malvern PA: Lea & Febiger; 1993.

Journal of Endourology. New York: May Ann Liebert; June 1992.

Journal of Urology. Vols. 147–149. Baltimore: Williams & Wilkins; 1992–93.

Massry, Textbook of nephrology, 2ed. Baltimore: Williams & Wilkins; 1989.

Novick, Stewart's operative urology, 2ed. Vols. 1–2. Baltimore: Williams & Wilkins; 1989.

Ostergard, Urogynecology and urodynamics, 3ed. Baltimore: Williams & Wilkins; 1991.

Your Medical Word Resource Publisher

We strive to provide you with the most up-to-date and accurate word references available. Your use of this word book will prompt new editions, which will be published as often as justified by updates and revisions. We welcome your suggestions for improvements, changes, corrections, and additions—whatever will make this **Stedman's** product more useful to you. Please use the postpaid card at the back of this book and send your recommendations to the Reference Division at Williams & Wilkins.

AAL
 anterior axillary line
Abbott
 A. IMx assay
 A. TDx monoclonal
 fluorescence
 polarization
 immunoassay
abdominal
 a. aortography
 a. compression belt
 a. muscle deficiency
 syndrome
 a. nephrectomy
 a. pressure
 a. testis
abdominoscrotal
 a. hydrocele
aberrant obturator vein
aberration
ablation
 cryogenic a.
 visual laser a.
abscess
 cavernosal a.
 cortical a.
 ischiorectal a.
 lacunar a.
 paranephric a.
 perinephric a.
 perirenal a.
 periureteral a.
 periurethral a.
 phlegmonous a.
 renal a.
 urachal a.
absorbable
 a. gelatin sponge
 a. suture
abuse
 substance a.

accessory
 a. adrenal
 a. vessel
acetaminophen
acetate
 buserelin a.
 cortisone a.
 cyproterone a. (CPA)
 desmopressin a.
 goserelin a.
 leuprolide a.
 medroxyprogesterone a.
 megestrol a.
 methylprednisolone a.
acetohydroxamic acid
acetowhite
 a. lesion
acetylcholine
acetylcholinesterase
acetylsalicylic acid
acid
 acetohydroxamic a.
 acetylsalicylic a.
 diethylenetriamine
 pentaacetic a. (DTPA)
 dimercaptosuccinic a.
 (DMSA)
 homovanillic a. (HVA)
 hyaluronic a.
 nalidixic a.
 p-amino-hippuric a.
 uric a.
 urine vanillylmandelic a.
 vanillacetic a. (VLA)
 vanillylmandelic a.
 (VMA)
acidosis
 hyperchloremic a.
 hyperchloremic
 metabolic a.
 renal tubular a.
acontractile detrusor

acorn-tipped catheter
acquired
   a. immunodeficiency
     syndrome (AIDS)
acrobystitis
acroposthitis
acrosin
ACTH
   adrenal corticotropic
   hormone
actinomycin D
actinomycosis
Active
   A. Living incontinence
     pads
   A. Living incontinence
     shield
acuminata, sing. acuminatum
   condylomata a.
acuminatum, pl. acuminata
   condyloma a.
acupuncture
acute
   a. focal bacterial
     nephritis (AFBN)
   a. interstitial nephritis
   a. nephritis
   a. nephrosis
   a. polycystic disease
   a. pyelonephritis
   a. scrotum
   a. urethritis
   a. vascular rejection
Acutrim
adapter
Addison syndrome
adductor
   a. brevis muscle
   a. longus muscle
adenocarcinoma
   clear cell a.
   prostatic a.
   renal a.
adenofibromyoma

adenoleiomyofibroma
adenoma
   cortical a.
   incidental a.
   Leydig cell a.
   nephrogenic a.
   Pick's tubular a.
   prostatic a.
   renal cortical a.
   testicular tubular a.
adenomatoid tumor
adenomatosis
   multiple endocrine a.
   type I (MEA-I)
   multiple endocrine a.
   type II (MEA-II)
adenomyosarcoma
adenosine triphosphate (ATP)
adherence
   bacterial a.
adhesion
   bacterial a.
   a. formation
   hepatic a.
   intraperitoneal a.
adhesive
   fibrin tissue a.
   Uro-Bond skin a.
adiphenine
adjuvant
   anesthesia a.
   a. chemotherapy
   a. drug therapy
   a. nephrectomy
   a. treatment
adnexal tumor
ADR
   Adriamycin
adrenal
   accessory a.
   a. cortex
   a. corticoadenoma
   a. corticotropic hormone
   (ACTH)

a. hirsutism
a. hyperplasia
a. rest
adrenal cortex
adrenalectomy
adrenal-like tissue
adrenocortical macrocyst
adrenogenital syndrome
Adriamycin (ADR)
Adson
A. clamp
A. forceps
adult polycystic disease (APCD)
advancement
Glenn-Anderson a.
meatal a.
adventitial
AERD
atheroembolic renal disease
aerocystoscope
aerocystoscopy
aeruginosa
Pseudomonas a.
AFBN
acute focal bacterial nephritis
AFP
alpha-fetoprotein
age
agenesis
renal a.

agent
antihypertensive a.
progesteronal a.
aggregation
erythrocyte a.
AIDS
acquired immunodeficiency syndrome
AIDS-related complex
Albarran
A. bridge
A. mechanism
A. reflecting bridge
A. test
albuginea
tunica a.
albumin
plasma a.
albuterol
Alcock's canal
alcohol
a. cooling bath
alcoholism
Alconefrin
aldesleukin
Proleukin a.
Aldoclor
Aldomet
Aldoril
aldosterone
aldosteronism
Aleo meter S-D2
Alexander elevator
alexandrite laser

NOTES

3

alfuzosin
Al-Ghorab
  A.-G. modification shunt
  A.-G. procedure
alkaloid
  indolalkylamine a.
alkaloids
  ergot a.
  Veratrum a.
alkalosis
Alken approach
allantoic cyst
allele
Allen's test
allergy
  latex a.
alligator forceps
Allis
  A. catheter
  A. clamp
  A. forceps
  A. tooth grasper
allograft
  kidney a.
  renal a.
  a. survival rate
allograft-mediated hypertension
alloplastic
  a. biomaterial
  a. prostatic bladder
allopurinol
allotransplantation
alpha
  a. blockade
  a. fetoprotein
alpha-1 blocker
alpha-fetoprotein (AFP)
Alpha I inflatable penile
  prosthesis
alpha-interferon therapy
Alport's syndrome
Alseroxylon-Alkavervir
alteration
  genetic a.

  molecular genetic a.
  nuclear matrix a.
alverine citrate
AMA inflatable cylinder
ambenonium chloride
ambiothermic
ambulation
ambulatory
  a. monitoring
  a. urodynamic
    monitoring
  a. urodynamics
amenorrhea
American
  A. Urological
    Association (AUA)
  A. Urological
    Association symptom
    index (AUA symptom
    index)
Ames Hemastix reagent strips
amifloxacin
Amin-Aid
amine
  aromatic a.
amine precursor uptake,
  decarboxylase (APUD)
4-Aminobiphenyl
aminoglutethimide
aminophylline
aminorex
amitriptyline
amnion
amodiaquine
amoxicillin
amphotericin B
ampicillin
Amplatz
  A. sheath
  A. superstiff guidewire
amputation
  penile a.

AMS
> AMS 742 artificial
> urinary sphincter
> AMS 761 artificial
> urinary sphincter
> AMS 791 artificial
> urinary sphincter
> AMS 792 artificial
> urinary sphincter
> AMS 800 artificial
> urinary sphincter
> AMS controlled
> expansion penile
> prosthesis cylinder
> (AMS CX penile
> prosthesis cylinder)
> AMS CX penile
> prosthesis cylinder
> AMS Hydroflex penile
> prosthesis
> AMS 600 malleable
> penile prosthesis
> AMS 700 penile
> prosthesis
> AMS Ultrex penile
> prosthesis

amsacrine (mAMSA)
amyloid nephrosis
analgesia
analgesic
> a. nephropathy

analysis
> contexture a.
> cost a.
> cytometric a.
> Diacyte DNA ploidy a.
> ploidy a.
> sequencing a.
> single strand
> conformation
> polymorphism a.
> spectrophotometric a.

analyzer
> Cell Soft 2000 semen a.
> Siemens Somatom DRH
> CT a.

Anandron
anaphylaxis
anaplastic
> a. tumor

anastalsis
> ureteroileourethral a.

anastomosis, pl. anastomoses
> Carrel aortic patch a.
> Daines-Hodgson a.
> dismembered a.
> end-to-end a.
> extravesical a.
> intravesical a.
> Lich-Gregoir a.
> mucosa-to-mucosa a.
> nondismembered a.
> Politano-Leadbetter a.
> right-angled end-to-
> side a.
> side-to-side a.
> tension-free a.
> transureteroureteral a.

NOTES

anastomosis *(continued)*
    two-layer a.
    ureterocolonic a.
    ureteroileal a.
    ureterosigmoid a.
    ureterotubal a.
    ureteroureteral a.
    vascular a.
    wide elliptical a.
anatomic stress incontinence
anatrophic
    a. nephrolithotomy
    a. nephroscopy
    a. nephrotomy
Ancef
anchoring suture
Anderson-Hynes
    A.-H. dismembered
      pyeloplasty
    A.-H. pyeloplasty
androblastoma
androgen
    a. blockade
    a. priming
    a. receptor
andrology
anejaculation
anemia
anephric
anesthesia adjuvant
aneurysm
    renal artery a.
    saccular a.
aneurysmectomy
angiogenesis
angiographic end hole catheter
angiography
    a. catheter
    digital subtraction a.
    subtraction a.
angioinfarction
angioma
angiomatoid tumor

Angiomed
    A. blue stent
    A. Puroflex stent
angiomyolipoma
angioneurectomy
angioneurotic hematuria
angioplasty
    a. balloon
    a. balloon catheter
    patch a.
    percutaneous
      transluminal a.
    percutaneous
      transluminal renal a.
      (PTRA)
angiotensin
angled dissecting forceps
angulation
anileridine
aniridia
anisotropine
ankylurethria
anorchia
anorchism
anorexia
antagonist
    hormone a.
antecubital arteriovenous
    fistula
antegrade
    a. approach
    a. cystography
    a. pyelogram
    a. urography
anterior
    a. approach
    a. axillary line (AAL)
    a. exenteration
    a. nephrectomy
    a. pelvic exenteration
    a. transabdominal
      approach
    a. urethra
antevesical hernia

antiandrogen
antibiotic
    broad-spectrum a.
    a. prophylaxis
antibody
    antisperm a.
    monoclonal a.
    OKT3 anti-T-cell a.
anti-BrDu
anticoagulant
anticoagulation
    a. therapy
antidepressant
antifol
    Baker's a.
antigen
    carcinoembryonic a.
    (CEA)
    ethylchlorformate
    polymerized a.
    immunobead-reacting a.
    Lewis X a.
    proliferating cell
    nuclear a. (PCNA)
    prostate-specific a. (PSA)
antihypertensive agent
anti-inhibin
antimicrobial
    a. prophylaxis
    a. therapy
antireflux
    a. Double-J stent
    a. procedure
antisense DNA inhibition

antisperm antibody
anuresis
anuretic
anuria
anuric
aortic
    a. patch
    a. punch
aortography
    abdominal a.
aortoiliac
aortorenal
    a. bypass
    a. reimplantation
aortotomy
apatite
    a. calculus
    carbonate a.
APCD
    adult polycystic disease
apellous
aperture
Aphrodyne
apical polar nephrectomy
aponeurosis
Appedrine
appendicovesicostomy
appendix
    a. epididymis
    a. testis
appliance
    external a.
    external cooling a.

NOTES

applicator
    multifire clip a.
    multiload occlusive
        clip a.
applier
    clip a.
    multiloaded clip a.
approach
    Alken a.
    antegrade a.
    anterior a.
    anterior
        transabdominal a.
    flank a.
    posterior a.
    posterior lumbar a.
    retroperitoneal a.
    thoracoabdominal a.
    thoracoabdominal
        extrapleural a.
    thoracoabdominal
        intrapleural a.
approximation
    tissue a.
approximator clamp
Apresoline
apron skin incision
APUD
    amine precursor uptake,
        decarboxylase
AquaMEPHYTON
Aramine
Arandel cell harvester
arcus
    a. tendineus fasciae
    a. tendineus fasciae
        pelvis
areflexia
    detrusor a.
areflexic bladder
argon
    a. beam coagulation
    a. beam coagulator
    a. laser

Army-Navy retractor
aromatic amine
Artane
arterialization
arteriogenic impotence
arteriograph
arteriography
    renal a.
arteriolar
arteriosclerosis
arteriovenous
    a. fistula
    a. malformation
    a. shunt
arteritis
    Takayasu's a.
artery
    bulbar a.
    deep a.
    hypogastric a.
    internal iliac a.
    internal pudendal a.
    umbilical a.
arthralgia
arthroplasty
artificial
    a. erection
    a. erection test
    a. kidney
    a. organ
    a. sphincter
    a. urinary sphincter
arylamine
AS
    A. 800 balloon
    A. 800 cuff
    A. 800 male bulbous
        urethra
    A. 800 pump
ASAP prostate biopsy needle
AS 800 balloon
ascending pyelonephritis
ascites
AS 800 cuff

Ashton
   A. briefs
   A. pants
ASI prostatic stent
Ask-Upmark
   A.-U. kidney
   A.-U. renal segment
aspartate transferase
aspermatism
aspermatogenic
   a. sterility
aspermia
aspiration
   a. and dissection tube
      percutaneous needle a.
   sperm a.
aspirator
   Cavitron ultrasonic a.
      (CUSA)
assay
   Abbott IMx a.
   Hybritech a.
   radioenzymatic a.
   Yang polyclonal a.
assessment
   outcome and process a.
   pain a.
   penile vascular
      function a.
ASSI laparoscopic electrode
assisted reproduction
Association
   American Urological A.
      (AUA)

association
   megacystis-megaureter a.
asthenospermia
asymptomatic
   a. bacteriuria
   a. mass
   a. urolithiasis
atelectasis
atenolol
atheroembolic renal disease
   (AERD)
atheromatous
atherosclerosis
atherosclerotic
   a. plaque
   a. renal artery stenosis
   a. stenosis
atonic bladder
ATP
   adenosine triphosphate
atraumatic
   a. clamp
   a. forceps
   a. grasper
   a. locking/grasping
      forceps
atresia
   follicular a.
   suprapubic cystotomy
      tract urethral a.
   urethral a.
atrial fibrillation
atrophy

NOTES

9

atropine
   a. methylnitrate
AUA
   American Urological
   Association
   AUA symptom index
augmentation
   a. cystoplasty
   ileocecocystoplasty
   bladder a.
   a. plaque
augmented bladder
autoantibody
autocystoplasty
autogenous
autoimmune
   a. deficiency syndrome
autolymphocyte therapy
autonomic
   a. dysreflexia

   a. nervous system
   a. neurogenic bladder
autoradiograph
autoregulation
Autosuture stapler
autotransplantation
   renal a.
autourethrography
Aventyl
axial image
azamethonium
azapetine
azathioprine
azoospermia
azotemia
AZQ
   diaziquone

Babcock
> B. clamp
> B. forceps

Babinski reflex
bacille Calmette-Guérin (BCG)
bacitracin
baclofen
bacteremia
bacterial
> b. adherence
> b. adhesion

bacteriuria
> asymptomatic b.
> catheter-associated b.

Bag
> Le B.

bag
> perfusate b.
> Petersen's b.

Baker's antifol
balanic
> b. hypospadias

balanitis
> b. circinata
> circinate b.
> b. circumscripta
>   plasmacellularis
> b. diabetica
> plasma cell b.
> trichomonal b.
> b. xerotica obliterans
>   (BXO)
> b. of Zoon

balanoblennorrhea
balanocele
balanoplasty
balanoposthitis
balanopreputial
balanorrhagia
balanorrhea
Balfour retractor

Balkan
> B. nephrectomy
> B. nephropathy

balloon
> angioplasty b.
> AS 800 b.
> b. catheter
> b. cystoscope
> b. dilation
> dissecting b.
> French Swan-Ganz b.
> Helmstein b.
> b. occlusion
> b. ureteral occlusion
> water displacing b.

Bamethan
band
> Lyon's ring-
>   constrictive b.

bandage
> suspensory b.
> T-b.

bar
> median b. of Mercier
> Mercier's b.

barbotage
Bard
> B. Biopty gun
> B. Biopty instrument

Bardex Foley catheter
barium
> b. enema

**Barrett-Donovan-Mayo
  artificial bladder**
base
> erythromycin b.

baseball stitch
basket
> Dormia retrieval b.
> Dormia stone b.
> Segura b.
> stone b.

basketing
Bassini operation
bath
    alcohol cooling b.
Baumrucker urinary
    incontinence clamp
BCG
    bacille Calmette-Guérin
    Calmette-Guérin bacillus
    TICE BCG
    BCG vaccine
BCR
    bulbocavernosus reflex
bead chain study
Beamer
    B. ejection stent
    B. injection stent system
Beckwith-Wiedemann
    syndrome
bed
    graft b.
bed-wetting
Beelith
Belladenal
belladonna
    tincture of b.
Bellergal-S
bell-shaped orifice
belt
    abdominal
        compression b.
Belt technique
Belzer machine
Benadryl
Benchekroun
    B hydraulic valve
    B pouch
bench surgical technique
benign
    b. mesothelioma of
        genital tract
    b. prostatic hyperplasia
        (BPH)

    b. prostatic hypertrophy
        (BPH)
Béniqué's sound
Bentson floppy-tipped
    guidewire
benzidine
benzodiazepine
benzphetamine
benztropine
benzydamine
BEP
    bleomycin, etoposide and
        cisplatin
Besnier-Boeck-Schaumann
    disease
beta
    growth factor b.
Betadine
beta-galactosidase
Betagan
beta-HCG
bethanechol
bethanidine
Bicitra
bicoudate catheter
bifid penis
bifurcation
bihisdin
bilabe
bilaminar embryonic disk
bilateral
    b. hydronephrosis
    b. incision
    b. lithotomy
    b. renal tumor
    b. renal vein thrombosis
    b. subcostal incision
    b. transabdominal
        incision
bilobar hyperplasia
bilobar hypertrophy
binder
    T-b.
binding

biochemical marker
Biodan Prostathermer
bioeffect
biofilm
BioGel P4
Bio-Gen
   B.-G. urine test strip
biologic
   b. response modifier
   therapy
   b. therapy
biological marker
biomaterial
   alloplastic b.
Biomydrin
biopsy
   brush b.
   cold cup b.
   digitally-guided b.
   b. forceps
   b. instrument
   needle b.
   renal b.
   Tru-Cut b.
   ultrasound-guided b.
Biopty
   B. cut needle
   B. gun
Biotel home screening test
biothesiometry
BIP biopsy instrument
biperiden
bipolar coagulating forceps
bisacodyl

bistable
Black Beauty ureteral stent
bladder
   alloplastic prostatic b.
   areflexic b.
   atonic b.
   augmented b.
   autonomic neurogenic b.
   Barrett-Donovan-Mayo
   artificial b.
   b. calculus
   b. cancer
   b. capacity
   b. carcinoma
   b. compliance
   cord b.
   b. exstrophy
   fasciculate b.
   b. fistula
   hypotonic b.
   ileal b.
   ileocecal b.
   ileocolonic b.
   b. inhibition
   low-compliance b.
   b. neck suspension
   b. neoplasm
   nervous b.
   neurogenic b.
   neuropathic b.
   b. neurosis
   orthotopic b.
   b. outflow obstruction
   b. outlet

NOTES

bladder *(continued)*
  b. outlet obstruction
  b. perforation
  b. pillar block
  b. pressure (BP)
  b. pressure sensor
  prosthetic b.
  pseudoneurogenic b.
  reflex neurogenic b.
  reflex neuropathic b.
  b. replacement
  b. stone
  b. substitution
  b. support
  b. tumor
  uninhibited
    neurogenic b.
  uninhibited overactive b.
  b. volume
  b. washing
blade
  Bovie b.
  malleable b.
blanket
  Gaymar water-
    circulating b.
bleeding
  b. control
  occult b.
bleomycin
**bleomycin, etoposide and
  cisplatin (BEP)**
Blocadren
block
  bladder pillar b.
  caudal b.
  nerve b.
blockade
  alpha b.
  androgen b.
blocker
  alpha-1 b.
  calcium entry b.

blood
  b. pressure (BP)
  b. transfusion
blue
  methylene b.
Bluemle pump
blunt
  b. dissection
  b. needle
blunt-tipped obturator
B-mode imaging
Boari
  B. bladder flap
  B. bladder flap
    procedure
  B. flap
  B. ureteral flap repair
Boari flap
Boari-Ockerblad flap
**Boden and Gibb tumor
  staging**
bodies
  Michaelis-Gutmann b.
body habitus
bombesin
bone
  b. marrow
    transplantation
  b. scan
Bonney test
bony spicule
Bookwalter
  B. retractor
  B. ring retractor
bore
  magnetic b.
Bosniak classification
botryoid
  b. sarcoma
bottle
  McGaw's plastic b.
bougie
  b. à boule
  wax-tipped b.

Bovie
B. blade
B. electrocautery
B. holder
bovis
Mycobacterium b.
bowel
b. forceps
b. obstruction
b. resection
bowel grasper
bowenoid papulosis
Bowen's disease
Bowman's capsule
Boyarsky symptom scoring system
Boyce
longitudinal nephrotomy of B.
Bozeman-Fritsch catheter
Bozeman operation
BP
bladder pressure
blood pressure
BPH
benign prostatic hyperplasia
benign prostatic hypertrophy
Braasch catheter
brachytherapy
interstitial b.
bradyspermatism
bradyuria

brain
b. metastasis
b. stem-sacral loop
b. stem-sacral loop bulbocavernosus reflex
branch
b. calculus
b. renal artery disease
branched
b. calculus
b. vascular graft
Braun stent
BrDu, BrdUrd
Bromodeoxyuridine
breakage
intracorporeal needle b.
Breakstone lithotriptor
breakthrough dose
breath
uremic b.
brequinar sodium
bretylium
Brevibloc
Brewer's infarcts
Bricker
B. operation
B. pouch
B. urinary diversion
bridge
Albarran b.
Albarran reflecting b.
briefs
Ashton b.

NOTES

briefs *(continued)*
  Holyoke b.
  Suretys incontinence b.
Bright's disease
brim
  pelvic b.
broad-spectrum antibiotic
Brodel's line
bromide
  methscopolamine b.
bromocriptine
Bromodeoxyuridine (BrDu, BrdUrd)
  B. cell kinetics
5-bromo-deoxyuridine
bromodiphenhydramine
brompheniramine
bropirimine
Brown dermatome
Bruel & Kjaer
  B. & K. scanner
  B. & K. 1846 ultrasound system
Brunschwig operation
brush
  b. biopsy
  b. catheter
buccal mucosal graft
Buck's fascia
bud
  ureteric b.
Budd-Chiari syndrome
Bugbee
  B. electrocautery
  B. electrode
bulbar
  b. artery
  b. urethral carcinoma
bulbocavernosus reflex (BCR)

bulbomembranous stricture
bulb-tipped retrograde ureterogram
bulb tip retrograde study
bulldog clamp
bullous
  b. edema
  b. edema vesicae
bundle
  neovascular b.
bupivacaine
  b. hydrochloride
bur
  Ultrasonic oscillating b.
Burch colposuspension
burden
  stone b.
Burnett's syndrome
burst
  respiratory b.
Buschke-Löwenstein tumor
buserelin
  b. acetate
buspirone
1-butanol
Butibel
butterfly needle
BXO
  balanitis xerotica obliterans
bypass
  aortorenal b.
  b. graft
  hepatorenal b.
  iliorenal b.
  mesenterorenal b.
  splenorenal b.

cable
    fiberoptic light c.
    internal fiberoptic c.
    light c.
cachexia
cadaver kidney
CAH
    congenital adrenal
    hyperplasia
Calcibind
Calcidrine syrup
calcification
calcite
calcitonin gene related peptide
    (CGRP)
calcium
    c. ATPase pump
    c. carbonate
    c. chloride
    c. entry blocker
    c. oxalate
    c. oxalate calculus
    c. oxalate nephrolithiasis
    c. oxaluria
    c. phosphate
    c. phosphate calculus
calculus, pl. calculi
    apatite c.
    bladder c.
    branch c.
    branched c.
    calcium oxalate c.
    calcium phosphate c.
    combination c.
    coral c.
    cystine c.
    decubitus c.
    dendritic c.
    c. disease
    encysted c.
    fusible c.
    indigo c.

    matrix c.
    midureteral c.
    c. migration
    mulberry c.
    nephritic c.
    oxalate c.
    pocketed c.
    preputial c.
    primary renal c.
    prostatic c.
    renal c.
    secondary renal c.
    staghorn c.
    struvite c.
    uric acid c.
    urinary c.
    vesical c.
    weddellite c.
    whewellite c.
Calcutript
    C. Electrohydraulic
    lithotriptor
    C. electrohydraulic
    lithotriptor
caldesmon
caliceal, calyceal
    c. diverticulum
    c. extension
    c. fornix
    c. infundibulum
calicectasis
calicectomy
calices (*pl. of* calix)
calicoplasty
calicotomy
caliectasis, calycectasis,
    calyectasis
caliectomy, calycectomy
calioplasty, calycoplasty,
    calyoplasty
caliorrhaphy, calyorrhaphy

caliotomy, calycotomy,
  calyotomy
calix, calyx, pl. calices
    c. puncture
Calmette-Guérin
    bacille C.-G. (BCG)
Calmette-Guérin bacillus
  (BCG)
calyceal (*var. of* caliceal)
calycectasis (*var. of*
  caliectasis)
calycectomy (*var. of*
  caliectomy)
calycoplasty (*var. of*
  calioplasty)
calycotomy (*var. of*
  caliotomy)
calyectasis (*var. of*
  caliectasis)
calyoplasty (*var. of*
  calioplasty)
calyorrhaphy (*var. of*
  caliorrhaphy)
calyotomy (*var. of* caliotomy)
calyx (*var. of* calix)
camera
    Olympus OTV-S2
    miniature c.
Camey
    C. enterocystoplasty
    C. enterocystoplasty
    urinary diversion
    C. procedure
Campbell
    C. sound
    C. technique
    C. trocar
Camwrap plastic covering
canal
    Alcock's c.
Cancer
cancer
    bladder c.

European Organization
  for Research and
  Treatment of c.
  (EORTC)
hypoechoic c.
c. screening
teratoma testicular c.
Candela Model MDL 2000
  laser
candidemia
candidiasis
cannula
    double-lumen
    irrigation c.
    Hasson c.
    Ramirez Silastic c.
cannulation
    ex vivo c.
Cantil
Cantwell epispadias repair
capacity
    bladder c.
    cystometric bladder c.
    functional bladder c.
    maximum bladder c.
    maximum cystometric c.
CAPD
    chronic ambulatory
    peritoneal dialysis
capistration
capnography
capnometry
capsular
    c. flap pyeloplasty
    c. penetration
capsulatum
    Histoplasma c.
capsule
    Bowman's c.
    c. flap technique
    prostatic c.
capsulotomy
    renal c.

captopril
   c. renography
captopril-DTPA
   c.-D. scanning
Cara-Klenz skin cleanser
carbachol
carbenicillin
carbonate
   c. apatite
   calcium c.
carboplatin
carboprost tromethamine
carbuncle
   kidney c., renal c.
**carcinoembryonic antigen
(CEA)**
carcinogenesis
   oncogene-induced c.
carcinoid tumor
carcinoma, pl. **carcinomas,
carcinomata**
   bladder c.
   bulbar urethral c.
   cervical c.
   clear cell c. of kidney
   embryonal c.
   embryonal testicular c.
   endometrial c.
   genitourinary c.
   germ cell c.
   medullary thyroid c.
   metastatic prostatic c.
   metastatic renal cell c.
   (MRCC)

   non-germ cell c.
   nonseminomatous
    testicular c.
   ovarian c.
   pancreatic c.
   pediatric c.
   penile c.
   primary transitional
    cell c.
   prostatic c.
   prostatic urethral
    transitional cell c.
   rectal c.
   renal c.
   renal cell c.
   renal pelvic c.
   renal pelvic transitional
    cell c.
   secondary metastatic c.
   sigmoid colon c.
   c. in situ (CIS)
   squamous cell c.
   stage B c.
   stage C c.
   supraglottic squamous
    cell c.
   testicular c.
   transitional cell c.
   ureteral c.
   urethral c.
   urothelial c.
   verrucous c.
   vulvar c.

NOTES

carcinomas (*pl. of*
carcinoma) (*pl. of* Glaxo
stain) (*pl. of* URYS 800
nerve stimulator) (*pl. of*
Gianturco metal urethral
stent)
carcinomata (*pl. of*
carcinoma) (*pl. of* Glaxo
stain) (*pl. of* URYS 800
nerve stimulator) (*pl. of*
Gianturco metal urethral
stent)
carcinosarcoma
 renal c.
cardiovascular disease
care
 home c.
 hospice c.
 palliative c.
C-arm fluoroscope
carmine
 indigo c.
carmustine
carphenazine
Carrel
 C. aortic patch
 C. aortic patch
  anastomosis
carrier
 ENDO-ASSIST
  disposable ligature c.
 Pereyra ligature c.
carteolol
Cartrol
caruncle
 urethral c.
cascara
CAS 200 image cytometer
Castleman disease
castrate
castration
 functional c.
catecholamine

catgut
 chromic c.
catheter
 acorn-tipped c.
 Allis c.
 angiographic end hole c.
 angiography c.
 angioplasty balloon c.
 balloon c.
 Bardex Foley c.
 bicoudate c., c. bicoudé
 Bozeman-Fritsch c.
 Braasch c.
 brush c.
 Clay-Adams PE-10 c.
 Clay-Adams PE-50 c.
 cobra c.
 conical c.
 Cope loop
  nephrostomy c.
 c. coudé
 c. à demeure
 de Pezzer c.
 double-lumen balloon c.
 Dowd prostatic balloon
  dilatation c.
 elbowed c.
 female c.
 Fogarty c.
 Foley c.
 French Cope loop
  nephrostomy c.
 French pigtail
  nephrostomy c.
 French Teflon
  pyeloureteral c.
 Gouley's c.
 c. guide
 Handi-Cath c. kit
 indwelling c.
 Inmed whistle tip
  urethral c.
 male c.
 Malecot c.

Malecot reentry c.
Millar c.
multifiber c.
mushroom c.
nephrostomy c.
olive-tipped c.
Pezzer c.
Phillips' c.
Porges c.
prostatic c.
pyeloureteral c.
red rubber c.
retrograde occlusion
 balloon c.
Robinson c.
self-retaining c.
Simplastic c.
spiral tip c.
stenting c.
Surgitek c.
Tandem thin-shaft
 transureteroscopic
 balloon dilatation c.
Tenckhoff c.
Texas style two-piece c.
Toronto-Western c.
Tracker c.
Tratner c.
ureteral occlusion
 balloon c.
Uro Max II high-
 pressure ureteral
 balloon dilatation c.

whistle-tip c.
Willscher c.
winged c.
catheter-associated bacteriuria
catheterization
 intermittent c.
 ureteral c.
 urinary c.
catheterize
cauda equina
 c. e. lesion
 c. e. syndrome
caudal
 c. block
 c. regression syndrome
cava
 vena c.
cavernitis
 fibrous c.
cavernosal abscess
cavernositis
cavernosogram
cavernosography
cavernosometry
 dynamic infusion c.
cavernosorum
 tunica albuginea
  corporum c.
cavernospongiosum shunt
cavernous
 c. hemangioma

NOTES

21

cavernous *(continued)*
   c. nerve-sparing
     prostatectomy
   c. vein
**Cavitron ultrasonic aspirator
  (CUSA)**
cavity
   nephrotomic c.
cavography
   vena c.
cavotomy
CBI
   continuous bladder
    irrigation
CCNU
   methyl C.
CE-24 needle
CEA
   carcinoembryonic antigen
Cecil procedure
cecocystoplasty
CEEA stapler
cefotaxime
cefpirome
cefpodoxime proxetil
ceftriaxone sodium
celiac
   c. tumor
Cell
   C. Analysis system
   C. Analysis system 200
    image cytometer (CAS
    200 image cytometer)
cell
   lymphokine-activated
    killer c. (LAK cell)
   natural killer c.
   oat c.
   proliferating c.
   c. proliferation
   schwannian spindle c.
   c. swelling
   transitional c.

**Cell Soft 2000 semen
  analyzer**
cellular infiltration
cellules
cellulitis
celomic epithelium
cephalad traction
cephalexin
cephalosporin
cerebral
   c. fluid shunt
   c. palsy
cerebral-brain stem circuit
cerebral-sacral loop
Cerespan
cervical
   c. carcinoma
   c. intraepithelial
    neoplasia (CIN)
cesium
CGRP
   calcitonin gene related
    peptide
chain
   obturator lymphatic c.
chancre
chancroid
channel
   sonotrode c.
charcoal
Chardonna-2
Charrière scale
chemoprophylaxis
chemosensitivity
chemotherapy
   adjuvant c.
   continuous infusion c.
   cytotoxic c.
   platinum-based
    consolidation c.
Cherney incision
Chester-Winter procedure
chest tube
chevron incision

Child's classification
chips
  prostatic c.
Chlamydia
  C. trachomatis
chlorambucil
chloride
  calcium c.
  oxybutynin c.
chlorisondamine
chlorohydrate
  linsidomine c.
chloroprocaine
chlorpheniramine
chlorphenoxamine
chlorpromazine
chlorprothixene
cholesterol
  radioactive c.
cholotriansene
chordee
choriocarcinoma
chorionic
choristoma
chromic
  c. catgut
  c. suture
chromocystoscopy
chromosome
  Y c.
chronic
  c. ambulatory peritoneal
    dialysis (CAPD)
  c. obstructive uropathy

  c. prostatitis
  c. pyelonephritis
chylocele
  parasitic c.
chyloderma
cigarette smoking
cimetidine
CIN
  cervical intraepithelial
    neoplasia
cineurography
Cipro
ciprofloxacin
  c. hydrochloride
circadian
circinate balanitis
circle needle
Circon-ACMI
  C.-ACMI uteroscope
Circon-ACMI lithotriptor
circuit
  cerebral-brain stem c.
  extracorporeal
    cardiopulmonary c.
circulation
  hepatic c.
circumcise
circumcision
  routine neonatal c.
  sleeve-type c.
cirrhosis
cirsocele
cirsoid

NOTES

CIS
   carcinoma in situ
CISCA
   cisplatin, cyclophosphamide
   and Adriamycin
cis, methotrexate and Velban
   (CMV)
cisplatin
cisplatin, cyclophosphamide
   and Adriamycin (CISCA)
cisplatinum
Citra Forte
citrate
   potassium c.
Citrobacter
   C. diversus
clamp
   Adson c.
   Allis c.
   approximator c.
   atraumatic c.
   Babcock c.
   Baumrucker urinary
    incontinence c.
   bulldog c.
   Cunningham urinary
    incontinence c.
   DeBakey c.
   Goldblatt c.
   Heaney c.
   Herrick c.
   Herrick kidney c.
   hilar c.
   Kelly c.
   kidney pedicle c.
   Kocher c.
   Microspike
    approximator c.
   microvascular c.
   mogen c.
   Moynihan c.
   noncrushing bowel c.
   occlusive c.
   partial-occlusion c.

   right-angle c.
   Satinsky c.
   straight mosquito c.
   tonsil c.
   tubing c.
   vascular c.
   Zeppelin c.
   Zipser penile c.
Clarke-Reich knot pusher
classification
   Bosniak c.
   Child's c.
   Kelami c.
   c. system
claw forceps
Clay-Adams
   C.-A. PE-10 catheter
   C.-A. PE-50 catheter
cleanser
   Cara-Klenz skin c.
   Rediwash skin c.
   UltraKlenz skin c.
clear
   c. cell adenocarcinoma
   c. cell carcinoma of
    kidney
   c. cell sarcoma
clearance
   kidney c.
cleavage plane
clidinium
CLIM computer program
clinical
   c. protocol
   c. trial
clip
   c. applier
   Heifitz c.
   Hulka c.
   metal c.
   silver c.
   titanium c.
   towel c.

cloacal
   c. exstrophy
   c. malformation
   c. membrane
   c. plate
Clomipramine
Clonidine suppression test
cloning
   molecular c.
clortermine
close suction drainage system
closure
   exstrophy c.
   muscularis tunnel c.
clot
   intraluminal c.
cloud phenomenon
clubbed penis
CMV
   cis, methotrexate and
   Velban
CO₂
   C. laser
   C. laser probe
coagulating electrode
coagulating forceps
coagulation
   argon beam c.
coagulator
   argon beam c.
coagulum pyelolithotomy
coarctation
cobalt-60

cobra catheter
Cochran-Mantel-Haenszel test
CODAS software
codeine
Cogentin
Cohen cross-trigonal
   reimplantation
Coherent Model 90-K laser
coil
   endoprostatic c.
   c. stent
colchicine
cold
   c. cup biopsy
   c. flushing
   c. knife
   c. knife endoureterotomy
   c. scissors
   c. storage
colectomy
Coley toxins
coli
   Escherichia c.
colic
   multiple recurrent
   renal c.
   renal c.
collagen
   glutaraldehyde cross-
   linked c. (GAX)
collagenase
collecting duct
collection system

NOTES

25

collector
    Misstique female
      external urinary c.
Colles' fascia
Collings
    C. electrosurgery knife
    C. knife
Collins
    C. indigo carmine
      solution
    C. intracellular
      electrolyte solution
    C. solution
colloid
colocystoplasty
colon conduit
coloproctostomy
color Doppler ultrasonography
colostomy
    end iliac c.
    juxta-anal c.
    loop transverse c.
    c. takedown
colosuspension
    Stamey c.
colovesical fistula
colpocleisis
    Latzko partial c.
colpocystocele
colpocystotomy
colpocystoureterotomy
colpogram
colposuspension
    Burch c.
colpoureterotomy
Colyte
combination calculus
combined ureterolysis
comorbidity
Compazine
compensatory testicular
   hypertrophy
complete duplication

complex
    AIDS-related c.
    exstrophy-epispadias c.
    histocompatibility c.
    nephroblastomatosis c.
    (NBC)
    oligohydramnios c.
    c. stone
compliance
    bladder c.
    vesical c.
complication
    postoperative c.
compression
    extrinsic c.
    spinal cord c.
compressor urethrae
computed tomography (CT)
Compu-void
concentric needle
condition
    intersex c.
conductance
    urethral electrical c.
conductivity
    electrical c.
conduit
    colon c.
    ileal c.
    Mitrofanoff c.
condyloma acuminatum
condylomata acuminata
Condylox
cone
    vaginal c. biopsy
congenital
    c. adrenal hyperplasia
    (CAH)
    c. hydrocele
    c. penile curvature
    c. penile deviation
    (CPD)
    c. renal mass
conical catheter

conjugated estrogen
connective tissue
connector
    Luer-Lok c.
    T c.
Connell stitch
Conn syndrome
Conray 60 contrast material
Conray 70 contrast material
construction
    vaginal c.
contexture analysis
contigen
continence
continent
    c. cutaneous diversion
    c. diversion
    c. urinary diversion
continuous
    c. bladder drainage
    c. bladder irrigation
    (CBI)
    c. catheter drainage
    c. hypothermic pulsatile
    perfusion
    c. infusion
    chemotherapy
contraceptive device
contractility
    normal detrusor c.
contracture
    Dupuytren's c.
    postinflammatory c.
contraindication

contrast
    c. enhancement
    c. medium
control
    bleeding c.
    fluoroscopic c.
    pain c.
    symptom c.
conus medullaris
Cook
    C. stent
    C. tissue morcellator
    C. urological trocar
coolant
cooling
    external c.
    homogenous c.
    ice c.
    immersion c.
    perfusion c.
    surface c.
    transarterial perfusion c.
    whole body c.
coordination
    R wave c.
Cope loop nephrostomy
    catheter
coral calculus
cord
    c. bladder
    spermatic c.
core-cut system
core temperature
Corgard

NOTES

corner suture
coronae
    papillomatosis c.
coronal sulcus
corpora cavernosa, sing. corpus
    cavernosum
corporeal
    c. veno-occlusive
        dysfunction
    c. venous occlusive
        dysfunction
corporoplasty
    modified Essed-
        Schroeder c.
corporotomy
corporovenous dysfunction
corpus cavernosum (*sing. of*
    corpora cavernosa)
corpus spongiosum
Corson
    C. needle
    C. needle electrosurgical
        probe
cortex
    adrenal c.
cortical
    c. abscess
    c. adenoma
corticoadenoma
    adrenal c.
corticoadrenal
    renal c.
cortisol
cortisone acetate
cost analysis
Co-trimoxazole
cough stress test
Coumadin
coumarin
Cowper's
    C. cyst
    C. gland
CPA
    cyproterone acetate

CPD
    congenital penile deviation
"crabs"
Cranley phleborrheograph
C-reactive protein
creatinine
creation
    Politano-Leadbetter
        tunnel c.
    tunnel c.
Crede maneuver
Crespo operation
Crile angle retractor
crista urethralis
criteria
    Foley c.
    morphometric c.
Crohn's disease
crossmatching
crus
cryogenic
    c. ablation
cryoprecipitate
cryoprecipitated plasma
cryopreservation
cryoprostatectomy
cryosurgery
cryptorchid
    c. testicle
    c. testis
cryptorchidectomy
cryptorchidism
cryptorchidopexy
cryptorchid testicle
cryptorchism
crystallization
crystalloid
CT
    computed tomography
cuff
    AS 800 c.
culdoplasty
    McCall c.

Culp
  C. pyeloplasty
  C. spiral flap
   pyeloplasty
culture
  tissue c.
  urine c.
**Cunningham urinary
 incontinence clamp**
cup
  vaginal fistula c.
cup-patch technique
current
  membrane c.
curvature
  congenital penile c.
curve
  Kaplan-Meier c.'s
  triphasic cystometric c.
curved
  c. dissecting forceps
  c. hemostat
  c. Maryland forceps
  c.-needle surgeon's knot
CUSA
  Cavitron ultrasonic
   aspirator
Cushing
  C. forceps
  C. syndrome
cushingoid
  c. facies
Cushing's disease

cutaneous
  c. ureterostomy
  c. urinary diversion
  c. vesicostomy
cutter
  rib c.
cutting
  c. electrode
  c. LR needle
cyanosis
cyclin
Cyclogyl
cyclooxygenase
  c. inhibitor
cyclopentamine
cyclophosphamide
  5-fluorouracil,
   Adriamycin and c.
   (FAC)
  vincristine, Adriamycin,
   and c. (VAC)
**cyclophosphamide, Velban,
 actinomycin-D, bleomycin,
 and platinum (VAB-VI)**
cyclosporine
cycrimine
cylinder
  AMA inflatable c.
  AMS controlled
   expansion penile
   prosthesis c. (AMS CX
   penile prosthesis
   cylinder)

NOTES

cylinder *(continued)*
    AMS CX penile
      prosthesis c.
        AMS controlled
          expansion penile
          prosthesis cylinder
      Ultrex c.
cyproterone acetate (CPA)
cyst
    allantoic c.
    Cowper's c.
    dermoid c.
    echinococcal c.
    glomerular c.'s
    hydatid c.
    inclusion c.
    junctional c.
    müllerian duct c.
    multilocular c.
    pilonidal c.
    renal c.
    tunic c.
    urachal c.
    urinary c.
cystalgia
cystathionine
cystauchenitis
cystauchenotomy
cystectasia, cystectasy
cystectomy
    partial c.
    radical c.
    salvage c.
    total c.
cystendesis
cystic
    c. dilation
    c. disease of renal
      medulla
    c. duct
    c. mass
    c. nephroma
    c. puncture
cystidoceliotomy

cystidolaparotomy
cystidotrachelotomy
cystine
    c. calculus
    c. lithiasis
    c. stone
cystinuria
cystistaxis
cystitis
    c. colli
    c. cystica
    emphysematous c.
    eosinophilic c.
    follicular c.
    c. glandularis
    honeymoon c.
    interstitial c.
Cystocath
cystocele
cystochromoscopy
cystodiaphanoscopy
cystodiverticulum
cystoenterocele
cystoepiplocele
cystogram
    micturating c.
    static c.
    voiding c.
cystography
    antegrade c.
cystojejunostomy
cystolith
cystolithectomy
cystolithiasis
cystolithic
cystolithotomy
cystolysis
cystometer
cystometric bladder capacity
cystometrogram
cystometrography
    voiding c.
cystometry
    gas c.

saline c.
screening c.
simultaneous urethral c.
voiding c.
water c.
cystopanendoscopy
cystoparalysis
cystopexy
cystophotography
cystoplasty
augmentation c.
Gil-Vernet ileocecal c.
human lyophilized
dura c.
cystoplegia
cystoproctostomy
cystoprostatectomy
cystoprostatourethrectomy
cystoptosis, cystoptosia
cystopyelitis
cystopyelonephritis
cystoradiography
cystorectostomy
cystorrhagia
cystorrhaphy
cystorrhea
cystoscope
balloon c.
Storz c.
Surgitek graduated c.
cystoscopic urography
cystoscopy
cystospasm
cystostaxis

cystostomy
trocar c.
c. tube
cystotome
cystotomy
suprapubic c.
cystotrachelotomy
cystoureteritis
cystoureterogram
cystoureterography
cystourethritis
cystourethrocele
cystourethrogram
voiding c. (VCUG)
cystourethrography
micturition c.
cystourethropexy
cystourethroscope
cystourethroscopy
dynamic c.
cytokeratin 8
cytokine therapy
Cytologic software
cytology
c. examination
cytomegalovirus
cytometer
CAS 200 image c.
Cell Analysis system
200 image cytometer
Cell Analysis system
200 image c. (CAS 200
image cytometer)
EPICS 752 flow c.

NOTES

cytometric analysis
cytometry
   deoxyribonucleic acid
    flow c.
   flow c.
   image c.
   static image DNA c.

cytopenia
cytophotometry
   static c.
cytotoxic chemotherapy
cytotoxicity

3-D
> 3-D computer
> reconstruction
> 3-D sonography

dacarbazine
Dacomed Catalyst VCD
Dacron graft
Daines-Hodgson anastomosis
Dale Foley catheter holder
damage
> tubular d.

Dantec
> D. 12-channel Urocolor
> Video System
> D. Etude system
> D. Menuet system
> D. rotating disk
> flowmeter
> D. UD5500 Mk2
> D. Urodyn 1000
> Flowmeter
> D. Urodyn 1000
> uroflowmeter

Dantrium
dantrolene
> d. sodium

Danubian endemic familial
nephropathy
dartos
> d. muscle
> d. pouch procedure

Datta procedure
DaVinci handle instrument
Davis
> D. interlocking sound
> D. intubated
> ureterotomy
> D. loop
> D. technique

DDAVP
> D. nasal spray

de
> d. novo
> d. Pezzer catheter

Deaner
Deaver retractor
deaza-aminopterin
DeBakey
> D. clamp
> D. forceps

debrisoquin
debulking
> percutaneous d.

decapacitation factor
decapsulation
> d. of kidney

decompensated neobladder
decompression
decortication
> renal cyst d.

decubitus calculus
deep
> d. artery
> d. dorsal vein
> d. trigone

de-epithelialization
defect
> intrapelvic filling d.

deferentectomy
deferentitis
deformity
> limb d.
> swan-neck d.

degloving
degree
> 120-d. lens
> 30-d. lens
> 70-d. lens

dehydroepiandrosterone (DHA)
> d. sulfate (DHAS)

dehydrogenase
> lactic d.
> lactic acid d. (LDH)

delay
    excretory d.
delta-5-pregnenolone
dementia
    dialysis d.
Demerol
dendritic calculus
Denis
    D. Browne pouch
Denonvilliers' fascia
density
    prostate-specific
      antigen d. (PSAD)
deoxydoxorubicin
deoxyepinephrine
deoxyribonucleic acid flow
  cytometry
Depo-Provera
Depostat
Depot
    Lupron D.
deprivation
    neoadjuvant
      hormonal d.
dermatitis
dermatome
    Brown d.
    Padgett d.
dermoid cyst
DES
    diethylstilbestrol
descensus
    d. aberrans testis
    d. paradoxus testis
descent
    perineal d.
    testicular d.
deserpidine
desipramine
desmopressin
    d. acetate
Desyrel
detection
    immunohistochemical d.

detorsion
detrusodetrusor facilitative
  reflex
detrusor
    acontractile d.
    d. activity index
    d. areflexia
    d. external sphincter
      dyssynergia
    d. hyperactivity
    d. hyperreflexia
    d. instability
    d. pressure
    d. sphincter dyssynergia
      (DSD)
    d. underactivity
detrusor-urethral dyssynergia
detrusosphincteric inhibitory
  reflex
detrusourethral inhibitory
  reflex
detumescence
devastated urethra
development
    embryologic d.
deviation
    congenital penile d.
      (CPD)
device
    contraceptive d.
    ErecAid vacuum
      erection d.
    implantable penile
      venous compression d.
    intrauterine d.
    linear stapling d.
    pneumatic
      compression d.
    Pos-T-Vac vacuum
      erection d.
    RigiScan d.
    "ring-type" rigidity
      measuring d.

Synergist vacuum
  erection d.
vacuum constriction d.
  (VCD)
vacuum erection d.
vacuum tumescence d.
VTU-1 vacuum
  erection d.
Wolf Piezolith 2300
  lithotripsy d.
Devine-Devine procedure
Devine hypospadias repair
devitalization
dexamethasone
Dexatrim
dexbrompheniramine
Dexedrine
Dexon suture
dextroamphetamine
dextropropoxyphene
DHA
  dehydroepiandrosterone
DHAS
  dehydroepiandrosterone
  sulfate
diabetes
  d. home screening test
  d. insipidus
  d. mellitus
diabetic impotence
Diacyte
  D. DNA ploidy analysis
Diafen

diagnosis
  noninvasive d.
  prenatal d.
  ultrasonic d.
diagnostic imaging evaluation
dialysate
dialysis
  d. access surgery
  chronic ambulatory
    peritoneal d. (CAPD)
  d. dementia
  d. disequilibrium
    syndrome
  d. encephalopathy
    syndrome
  extracorporeal d.
  peritoneal d.
diaminedichloroplatinum
diamond jaw needle holder
diamorphine
dianhydrogalactiol
diaphragm
  urogenital d.
diarrhea
diary
  voiding d.
Diasonics DRF ultrasound
  unit
diastematomyelia
diatrizoate
  meglumine d.
diazepam
diaziquone (AZQ)
diclofenac sodium

NOTES

dicyclomine
Didrex
didymalgia
didymitis
dietary purine
diethylenetriamine pentaacetic
acid (DTPA)
diethylenetriaminepentaacetic
acid renography (DTPA
renography)
diethylpropion
diethylstilbestrol (DES)
Dietrol
differential
  d. renal function test
  d. ureteral
  catheterization test
differentiation
  genital d.
  gonadal d.
  sexual d.
diffractometry
  x-ray d.
diffuse
  d. mesangial
  proliferation
Diflucan
DIF-test
  direct immunofluorescence
  test
digestion
digital
  d. rectal examination
  (DRE)
  d. subtraction
  angiography
digitally-guided biopsy
Dignity incontinence pants
digoxin
dihydroergotoxine
dihydroxyphenylalanine
  (DOPA)
Dilamezinsert instrument
dilating set

dilation
  balloon d.
  cystic d.
  tract d.
  transurethral balloon d.
  urethral d.
dilator
  120 Fr balloon d.
  Kollmann's d.
  Nottingham ureteral d.
  Optilume prostate
  balloon d.
  prostate balloon d.
  vessel d.
  Walther d.
dildo, dildoe
diltiazem
dimenhydrinate
dimercaptosuccinic
  d. acid (DMSA)
  d. acid scintigraphy
  (DMSA scintigraphy)
dimethylsulfoxide
dimethyl sulfoxide
dimethyltriazenoimidazole-
  carboxamide (DTIC)
Diodrast
dioxethedrin
diphallia
diphallus
diphemanil
direct
  d. immunofluorescence
  test (DIF-test)
  d. inguinal hernia
  d. manipulation
Direx Tripter X-1 lithotriptor
DISA
  DISA electromyography
  DISA needle electrode
  DISA 5500 urograph
disease
  acute polycystic d.

adult polycystic d. (APCD)
Besnier-Boeck-Schaumann d.
Bowen's d.
branch renal artery d.
Bright's d.
calculus d.
cardiovascular d.
Castleman d.
Crohn's d.
Cushing's d.
cystic d. of renal medulla
Dupuytren's d.
end-stage d.
infantile polycystic d. (IPCD)
inflammatory bowel d.
intramural atheromatous d.
Marion's d.
metabolic stone d.
microcystic d. of renal medulla
minimal-change d.
nil d.
Ormond's d.
Paget's d.
Parkinson's d.
Peyronie's d.
polycystic kidney d.
renal arterial occlusive d.
renal cystic d.
sexually transmitted d. (STD)
stone d.
suprahilar d.
Takayasu's d.
upper tract d.
van Buren's d.
venereal d.
von Hippel-Lindau d.
Weber-Christian d.

disintegration
  endoscopic stone d.
disjoined pyeloplasty
disk
  bilaminar embryonic d.
dismembered
  d. anastomosis
  d. pyeloplasty
dismutase
  superoxide d.
disodium edetate
displacement
disruption
dissecting balloon
dissection
  blunt d.
  extended obturator node and iliopsoas node d.
  intracapsular d.
  limited obturator node d.
  d. margin
  plane of d.

NOTES

dissection *(continued)*
    preadventitial d.
    d. scissors
    sharp d.
    spontaneous d.
dissemination
    metastatic d.
distal
    d. ureterectomy
    d. venous plexus
distortion
distribution
    node d.
Ditropan
Diupres
diuresis
    post-obstructive d.
diuretic
Diutensen-R
diversion
    Bricker urinary d.
    Camey enterocystoplasty
      urinary d.
    continent d.
    continent cutaneous d.
    continent urinary d.
    cutaneous urinary d.
    Duke pouch cutaneous
      urinary d.
    fecal d.
    Gil-Vernet ileocecal
      cystoplasty urinary d.
    hemi-Kock urinary d.
    ileal conduit urinary d.
    ileocolic urinary d.
    Khafagy modified
      ileocecal cystoplasty
      urinary d.
    Kock pouch cutaneous
      urinary d.
    Mainz pouch cutaneous
      urinary d.
    Studer reservoir
      urinary d.

    supravesical urinary d.
    urinary d.
diverticula (*pl. of*
  diverticulum)
diverticulectomy
    urethral d.
    vesical d.
diverticulitis
    sigmoid d.
diverticulum, pl. **diverticula**
    caliceal d.
    noncommunicating d.
    urethral d.
    vesical d.
DMSA
    dimercaptosuccinic acid
    DMSA scintigraphy
DNA
docusate sodium
dolphin grasping forceps
dolphin-type atraumatic
  forceps
dome
Domperidone
donation
    organ d.
Donnagel
Donnatal
donor
donovanosis
DOPA
    dihydroxyphenylalanine
dopamine
Dopar
Doppler
    Intradop
      intraoperative D.
    D. probe
    pulsed D.
    D. QAD-1
    D. Quantum color flow
      system
    D. ultrasonography

Dormia
  D. retrieval basket
  D. stone basket
Dornier
  D. HM3 lithotriptor
  D. HM4 lithotriptor
  D. MFL 5000 urological
    workstation
dorsal
  d. lithotomy position
  d. lumbotomy incision
  d. nerve of penis
  d. slit
dose
  breakthrough d.
dose-response
double
  d. cuff AMS 800
    urinary sphincter
  d. penis
double-J
  d.-J. stent
  d.-J. Surgitek catheter
    stent
  d.-J. ureteral stent
double-lumen
  d.-l. balloon catheter
  d.-l. irrigation cannula
doubling time
**Dowd prostatic balloon
  dilatation catheter**
downstaging
  hormonal d.
Down syndrome

doxazosin
doxepin
doxorubicin
doxycycline monohydrate
Doyen rib elevator
drain
  Jackson-Pratt d.
  Penrose d.
  suction d.
drainage
  continuous bladder d.
  continuous catheter d.
  gravity-dependent d.
  percutaneous d.
  tidal d.
"drainpipe"
  frozen "drainpipe"
Drake Uroflometer
drape
  Lingeman 3 in 1
    procedure d.
  Lingeman TUR d.
  O'Conor d.
  surgical d.
DRE
  digital rectal examination
dribble
  postmicturition d.
dribbling
driver
  laparoscopic needle d.
  needle d.
droperidol

NOTES

drug
    d. carrier system
    nonsteroidal anti-
      inflammatory d.
      (NSAID)
    parasympatholytic d.'s
    parasympathomimetic d.'s
    psychotropic d.
    d. resistance
    d. therapy
    vasoactive d.
DSD
    detrusor sphincter
    dyssynergia
DTIC
    dimethyltriazenoimidazole-
    carboxamide
DTPA
    diethylenetriamine
    pentaacetic acid
    DTPA renography
duck-bill forceps
ducreyi
    Haemophilus d.
duct
    collecting d.
    cystic d.
    excretory d.
    mesonephric d.
    müllerian d.
    Skene's d.
    wolffian d.
ductal system
ductule efferentes
Duke
    D. pouch
    D. pouch cutaneous
      urinary diversion
dumbbell-shaped calyceal
  extension
duplication
    complete d.
    incomplete d.
    renal d.

Dupuytren's
    D. contracture
    D. disease
    D. hydrocele
Duraphase penile prosthesis
dye
    d. laser
    d. sham intrarenal
    lesion
Dynaflex penile prosthesis
dynamic
    d. cystourethroscopy
    d. infusion
    cavernosometry
dysfunction
    corporeal veno-
      occlusive d.
    corporeal venous
      occlusive d.
    corporovenous d.
    erectile d.
    geriatric voiding d.
    human erectile d.
    neuropathic d.
    urodynamic d.
dysfunctional voiding
dysgenesis
    gonadal d.
dysgerminoma
dyspareunia
dysplasia
    fibrous d.
    renal duplication with
      segmental renal d.
    segmental renal d.
dysreflexia
    autonomic d.
dysspermatogenic sterility
dyssynergia
    detrusor external
      sphincter d.
    detrusor sphincter d.
    (DSD)
    detrusor-urethral d.

vesical external
  sphincter d. (VSD)
vesicosphincteric d.
dystopia
  d. transversa externa
  testis

  d. transversa interna
  testis
dysuria
dysuric

NOTES

E_1
prostaglandin E.
Eastern Cooperative Oncology
 Group (ECOG)
Ebbehoj procedure
echinococcal cyst
echinococcosis
Echinococcus
echocardiography
echogenicity
echo pattern
ECOG
 Eastern Cooperative
 Oncology Group
 ECOG performance
 status scale
ectoderm
ectopia
 e. testis
 transverse testicular e.
 e. vesicae
ectopic
 e. adrenal rest
 e. testis
 e. ureter
 e. ureterocele
EDAP LT.01 lithotriptor
edema
 bullous e.
 bullous e. vesicae
edetate
 disodium e.
EDRF
 endothelium-derived
 relaxing factor
edrophonium
EEA stapler
effect
 hypothermic e.
 intracellular flush e.
 mitrogenic e.
 normothermic e.

placebo e.
preservation times e.
rormothermic e.
efferentes
 ductule e.
efficacy
Eisenberger technique
ejaculatio
 e. deficiens
 e. praecox
 e. retardata
ejaculation
 premature e.
ejaculatory
 e. duct obstruction
 e. impotence
elastica interna
Elavil
elbowed catheter
electrical conductivity
electric tissue morcellator
electrocardiogram
electrocautery
 Bovie e.
 Bugbee e.
 light e.
 e. resection
electrocystography
electrode
 ASSI laparoscopic e.
 Bugbee e.
 coagulating e.
 cutting e.
 DISA needle e.
 flat spatula e.
 Greenwald Control Tip
 cystoscopic e.
 hook e.
 hook tip laparoscopic e.
 J hook tip
 laparoscopic e.
 knife e.

electrode *(continued)*
    loop-tipped e.
    needle e.
    needle tip
      laparoscopic e.
    pencil-tipped e.
    reusable laparoscopic e.
    right-angle e.
    spatula tip
      laparoscopic e.
    spoon tip
      laparoscopic e.
    three-quarter circle e.
electroejaculation
    rectal probe e.
electroejaculator
electrohydraulic
    e. lithotripsy
    e. lithotriptor
    e. lithotriptor probe
electrolyte
    e. flush solution
electromechanical impactor (EMI)
electromyography
    DISA e.
    rhabdosphincter e.
electronic recording nappies
electron microscopy
electrosurgery
electrosurgical
    e. curved scissors
    e. monopolar spatula
      probe
    e. needle
    e. probe
    e. scissors
    e. spatula
    e. unit
elephantiasis
    e. scroti
elevator
    Alexander e.
    Doyen rib e.

eleventh
    e. rib flank incision
    e. rib transperitoneal
      incision
Ellik evacuator
elusive ulcer
emasculation
embolism
    pulmonary e.
embolization
embryologic development
embryology
embryoma
    e. of the kidney
embryonal
    e. carcinoma
    e. testicular carcinoma
Emcyt
emepronium
EMI
    electromechanical impactor
emission
emotional support
emphysematous cystitis
empyocele
enanthate
    testosterone e.
en bloc technique
encapsulation
    tumor e.
encasement
    ureteral e.
encysted calculus
end
    e. iliac colostomy
    e. stoma
endarterectomy
    e. knife
end-end stapler
end-fire transrectal probe
ENDO-ASSIST
    E.-A. disposable
      atraumatic grasping
      forceps

E.-A. disposable
hemostat
E.-A. disposable ligature
carrier
E.-A. disposable needle
holder
E.-A. reusable knot
pusher
endocast
EndoClip
endocrine
  e. screening
  e. system
  e. therapy
endocystitis
endogenous pyrogen
EndoGIA 30 stapler
EndoGIA 60 stapler
Endo-GIA stapler
endoligature
endometrial carcinoma
Endopath 30 stapler
Endopath 60 stapler
endoprostatic coil
endopyelotomy
endorectal probe
endoscope
  flexible e.
  semirigid e.
endoscopic
  e. alligator forceps
  e. flowprobe
  e. fulguration

  e. scissors
  e. stone disintegration
endoscopy
Endoshears
endosnare
Endostapler
Endotek-Ultra Urodynamics
  System
endothelin
endothelin-1
endothelin-3
endothelium
endothelium-derived
  e.-d. relaxing factor
    (EDRF)
endoureteral ultrasound
  sonography
endoureterotomy
  cold knife e.
endourologic
endourology
endoypelotomy
Endrate
end-stage disease
end-to-end
  e.-t.-e. anastomosis
  e.-t.-e. branch
    reanastomosis
end-to-side reimplantation
Enduronyl
enema
  barium e.
  Fleet e.
enflurane

NOTES

electrovaporization

45

engraftment
enhancement
  contrast e.
enolase
  neuron-specific e. (NSE)
enoxacin
Ensure
  E. Plus
enteral nutrition
enteritis
  radiation e.
enterocutaneous fistula
enterocystocele
enterocystoplasty
  Camey e.
  sigmoid e.
enteroenterostomy
  two-layer e.
enteropathy
enterotomy
  inadvertent e.
  longitudinal e.
enterourethrostomy
enterovesical fistula
enterovesicoplasty
entoderm
entrapment
  e. sack
  e. sack introducer
entry site
enucleation
enuresis
  nocturnal e.
EORTC
  European Organization for
  Research and Treatment of
  Cancer
eosin
eosinophilic cystitis
eosinophiluria
EPICS 752 flow cytometer
epicystotomy
epidermal growth factor

epidermidis
  Staphylococcus e.
epididymectomy
epididymidectomy
epididymis, pl. epididymides
  appendix e.
epididymisoplasty
epididymitis
epididymo-orchitis
epididymoplasty
epididymotomy
epididymovasectomy
epididymovasostomy
epinephrine
epipodophyllotoxin
epirubicin
epispadia
epispadiac orifice
epispadial
epispadias
  subsymphyseal e.
epistaxis
  renal e.
epithelium
  celomic e.
  nonkeratinizing
    squamous e.
  transitional e.
EPL
  extracorporeal piezoelectric
  lithotripsy
Epodyl
epoophoron
ErecAid
  E. system
  E. vacuum erection
    device
  E. vacuum system
erectile
  e. dysfunction
  e. potency
erection
  artificial e.
  artificial e. test

penile e.
   vacuum constriction e.
ergot alkaloids
erosion
erythrocyte aggregation
erythrocytosis
erythromycin base
erythroplasia
   e. of Queyrat
   Zoon's e.
erythropoietin
   human recombinant e.
Escherichia coli
Esimil
esmolol
essential hematuria
esthesioneuroblastoma
estradiol
   ethinyl e.
Estradurin
estramustine
   e. phosphate
   e. phosphate sodium
estrogen
   conjugated e.
ESWL
   extracorporeal shock wave
   lithotripsy
ethanolamine oleate
Ethaquin
ethaverine
Ethicon trocar
ethinyl estradiol
ethopropazine

ethylchlorformate polymerized
   antigen
etiology
etoposide
EU
   excretory urography
Eulexin
European Organization for
   Research and Treatment of
   Cancer (EORTC)
Eutonyl
evacuator
   Ellik e.
evaluation
   diagnostic imaging e.
   follow-up e.
   medical e.
   metabolic e.
   presurgical medical e.
   sexual e.
   videourodynamic e.
eviration
evisceration
   total abdominal e.
   (TAE)
evoked potential
Ewing's sarcoma
ex
   e. vivo
   e. vivo cannulation
examination
   cytology e.
   digital rectal e. (DRE)
   rectal e.

NOTES

excision
excretion
   urinary e.
excretory
   e. delay
   e. duct
   e. urography (EU)
exenteration
   anterior e.
   anterior pelvic e.
   pelvic e.
   posterior e.
   posterior pelvic e.
   supralevator e.
   total pelvic e.
exercise
   Kegel pelvic muscle e.
Exna
expanding retroperitoneal
  hematoma
expression
   tissue-specific gene e.
exsanguination
exstrophy
   e. of the bladder
   bladder e.
   cloacal e.
   e. closure
   vesical e.
exstrophy-epispadias complex
extended
   e. left subcostal incision
   e. obturator node and
     iliopsoas node
     dissection
   e. pyelotomy
extensibility
   penile e.
extension
   caliceal e.
   dumbbell-shaped
     calyceal e.

external
   e. anal sphincter muscle
   e. appliance
   e. beam radiation
     therapy
   e. cooling
   e. cooling appliance
   e. fascia
   e. spermatic vein
   e. urethrotomy
   e. vacuum therapy
extracapsular
   e. tumor
extracorporeal
   e. cardiopulmonary
     circuit
   e. dialysis
   e. partial nephrectomy
   e. piezoelectric
     lithotripsy (EPL)
   e. preservation
   e. renal preservation
   e. repair
   e. shock wave
     lithotripsy (ESWL)
   e. shock wave
     lithotriptor
   e. surgery
extraction
extraprostatitis
extrarenal mass
extravasation
extraversion
   urinary e.
extravesical
   e. anastomosis
   e. ureterolysis
extrinsic compression
eyepiece

F

F2 focal point
FAC
   5-fluorouracil, Adriamycin
    and cyclophosphamide
faceplate
facies
   cushingoid f.
   Potter f.
factor
   decapacitation f.
   endothelium-derived
    relaxing f. (EDRF)
   epidermal growth f.
   müllerian inhibiting f.
   nuclear roundness f.
   prognostic f.
   tumor necrosis f. (TNF)
Fader
   F. Tip ureteral stent
failure
   irradiation f.
   kidney f.
   renal f.
   f. to thrive
   treatment f.
familial
   f. juvenile
    nephrophthisis
   f. nephrosis
   f. pheochromocytoma
fan retractor
fan-type laparoscopic retractor
fascia
   Buck's f.
   Colles' f.
   Denonvilliers' f.
   external f.
   fusion f.
   f. of Gerota
   Gerota's f.
   lumbosacral f.
   rectal f.
   renal f.
   Scarpa's f.
fasciae
   arcus tendineus f.
fasciculate bladder
fasciitis
   necrotizing f.
fat
   perivesical f.
fatigue
   suture f.
febrile
   f. morbidity
fecal
   f. diversion
   f. spillage
fecaluria
female catheter
femoral triangle
fentanyl
Fenwick-Hunner ulcer
ferritin
fertility
   f. status
fertilization
   in vitro f.
fetoprotein
   alpha f.
Feulgen
   F. reaction
   F. staining
fiberoptic light cable
fiber optics
fiberscope
fiberTome system
fibrillation
   atrial f.
fibrin
   f. tissue adhesive
fibrinogen
fibrodysplastic
fibroelastic tissue

fibroelastosis
fibroma
fibromatosis
  penile f.
fibromuscular hyperplasia
fibronectin
fibroplasia
  intimal f.
  medial f.
  perimedial f.
fibrosarcoma
fibrosis
  idiopathic
    retroperitoneal f.
  periureteral f.
  retroperitoneal f.
  tubulointerstitial f.
fibrous
  f. cavernitis
  f. dysplasia
figure-of-eight suture
filarial hydrocele
filiform tip
filter
  Greenfield f.
  suprarenal Greenfield f.
finasteride
Finochietto retractor
first-stage repair
Fisher exact test
fistula, pl. **fistulae, fistulas**
  antecubital
    arteriovenous f.
  arteriovenous f.
  bladder f.
  colovesical f.
  enterocutaneous f.
  enterovesical f.
  forearm graft
    arteriovenous f.
  gastric f.
  genitourinary f.
  ileosigmoid f.
  ileovesical f.

intestinal f.
perineal urinary f.
rectourethral f.
rectovesical f.
renogastric f.
spermatic f.
thigh graft
  arteriovenous f.
ureterocolic f.
ureterocutaneous f.
ureterovaginal f.
urethrocavernous f.
urethrorectal f.
urethrovaginal f.
urinary f.
urinary umbilical f.
urogenital f.
vasocutaneous f.
vesical f.
vesicocolic f.
vesicocutaneous f.
vesicointestinal f.
vesico-ovarian f.
vesicorectal f.
vesicosalpingovaginal f.
vesicouterine f.
vesicovaginal f.
vesicovaginorectal f.
five-port "fan" placement
fixed ring retractor
FK 506
Flagyl
flank
  f. approach
  f. incision
  f. mass
  f. position
flap
  Boari f.
  Boari bladder f.
  Boari-Ockerblad f.
  foreskin f.
  island pedicle f.
  Martius f.

myocutaneous f.
onlay island f.
Scardino f.
surgical f.
u-shaped skin f.
ventrum penis f.
FLASH
flat low-angle shot
FLASH pulse sequence
flat
f. low-angle shot
(FLASH)
f. spatula electrode
Fleet enema
flexible
f. endoscope
f. nephroscope
f. nephroscopy
f. tip guide wire
f. ureteropyeloscopy
Flexi-Flate
F.-F. II penile prosthesis
F.-F. I penile prosthesis
flexion
Flexirod penile prosthesis
flip-flap
Mathieu-Horton-
Devine f.-f.
Florida pouch
Floropryl
flow
f. cytometric study
f. cytometry
plasma f.

f. rate
turbulent f.
Flowmeter
Dantec Urodyn 1000 F.
flowmeter
Dantec rotating disk f.
laser Doppler f.
flowprobe
endoscopic f.
Floxin
fluconazole
fluid
irrigating f.
flumazenil
fluorodeoxyuridine
fluoroquinolone
fluoroscope
C-arm f.
fluoroscopic
f. control
f. monitoring
fluorouracil
5-fluorouracil (5-FU)
**5-fluorouracil, Adriamycin and
cyclophosphamide (FAC)**
fluorourodynamics
fluoxymesterone
fluphenazine
flushing
cold f.
flutamide
focal
**focal-segmental
glomerulosclerosis**

NOTES

ʃ

51

focused shock wave
Fogarty catheter
Foley
    F. catheter
    F. criteria
    F. operation
    F. Y-plasty pyeloplasty
    F. Y-V plasty
follicle-stimulating hormone
  (FSH)
follicular
    f. atresia
    f. cystitis
follow-up evaluation
forceps
    Adson f.
    Allis f.
    atraumatic f.
    atraumatic
      locking/grasping f.
    Babcock f.
    biopsy f.
    bowel f.
    claw f.
    curved dissecting f.
    curved Maryland f.
    Cushing f.
    DeBakey f.
    dolphin grasping f.
    dolphin-type
      atraumatic f.
    duck-bill f.
    ENDO-ASSIST
      disposable atraumatic
      grasping f.
    endoscopic alligator f.
    Gerald f.
    grasping f.
    hook f.
    jeweler's f.
    Lalonde hook f.
    Mazzariello-Caprini f.
    Millin f.
    packing f.
    perforating f.
    Potts f.
    radial jaw bladder
      biopsy f.
    Randall stone f.
    Semken tissue f.
    spoon f.
    stone f.
    straight Maryland f.
    toothed f.
    traumatic grasping f.
Forder retractor
forearm graft arteriovenous
  fistula
foreign body reaction
foreskin
    f. flap
fork
    stimulation f.
formation
    adhesion f.
    median bar f.
    pseudoaneurysm f.
fornix
    caliceal f.
Foroblique resectoscope
Fortaz
Foscarnet
fossa
    f. navicularis
    prostatic f.
Fournier's gangrene
four-port "diamond" placement
Fowler-Stephens
    F.-S. maneuver
    F.-S. orchiopexy
    F.-S. procedure
Fr (Fr)
    Fr
fraction
    plasma protein f.
fragment
    residual f.

fragmentation
  stone f.
  ultrasonic f.
Fraley syndrome
Frazier suction tube
120Fr balloon dilator
free radical scavenger
French
  F. Cope loop
    nephrostomy catheter
  F. double-J ureteral
    stent
  F. introducer set
  F. pigtail nephrostomy
    catheter
  F. Swan-Ganz balloon
  F. Teflon pyeloureteral
    catheter
frenulum
frequency-urgency-pain
  syndrome
friable
frozen
  f. "drainpipe"
  f. section
FSH
  follicle-stimulating hormone
5-FU
  5-fluorouracil

fulguration
  endoscopic f.
function
  kidney f.
  renal f.
  sexual f.
functional
  f. bladder capacity
  f. castration
  f. profile length
fungal infection
Fungizone
funguria
funicular hydrocele
funiculopexy
Furacin
Furlow cylinder inserter
Furlow-Fisher modification of
  Virag 1 operation
furosemide
fusible calculus
fusiform
fusion
  f. fascia
  urethrohymenal f.
Fusobacterium

NOTES

GAGUA
glycosaminoglycans uronate
gallium scan
gamete intrafallopian transfer (GIFT)
gamma-glutamyl-transpeptidase
gamma-interferon
ganglia
intramural g.
ganglioneuroma
gangliosides
gangrene
Fournier's g.
gantry
gap
g. junction
underwater spark g.
Gardnerella vaginalis
gas cystometry
gastric
g. fistula
g. neobladder
gastrocystoplasty
gastroepiploic blood vessel
Gastrografin
G. GI series
gastrostomy
Stamm g.
GAX
glutaraldehyde cross-linked collagen
GAX-collagen
Gaymar water-circulating blanket
Gazayerli
G. knot pusher
Gelfoam
gene
tumor suppressor g.
genetic
g. alteration
g. predisposition

genital differentiation
genitalia
genitofemoral nerve
genitourinary
g. carcinoma
g. fistula
g. neoplasm
g. prolapse
g. tract
gentamicin
gentian violet
Gerald forceps
Gerhardt table
geriatrics
geriatric voiding dysfunction
germ
g. cell carcinoma
g. cell tumor
Gerota
fascia of G.
Gerota's fascia
GFR
glomerular filtration rate
G.F.S. Mark II inflatable penile prosthesis
GIA
G. instrument
G. stapler
Gianturco metal urethral stent, pl. carcinomas, carcinomata
Gibson incision
Gibson-type incision
GIFT
gamete intrafallopian transfer
Gilchrist procedure
Gil-Vernet
G.-V. ileocecal cystoplasty

Gil-Vernet *(continued)*
　　G.-V. ileocecal
　　　cystoplasty urinary
　　　diversion
　　G.-V. operation
　　G.-V. procedure
　　G.-V. retractor
　　G.-V. technique
Gittes technique
gland
　　Cowper's g.
glansplasty
　　meatal advancement
　　　and g. (MAGPI)
glanuloplasty
Glaxo stain, pl. **carcinomas,
carcinomata**
Gleason
　　G. cancer grade
　　G. grade
　　G. score
　　G. staging system
gleet
gleety
Glenn-Anderson advancement
Glidewire guide wire
globulin
　　sex hormone binding g.
　　　(SHBG)
glomerular
　　g. cysts
　　g. filtration rate (GFR)
glomerulation
glomeruli (*pl. of* glomerulus)
glomerulitis
glomerulonephritis
　　mesangial proliferative g.
　　recurrent focal
　　　sclerosing g.
glomerulopathy
glomerulosa
　　zona g.

glomerulosclerosis
　　focal-segmental g.
glomerulus, pl. **glomeruli**
glucocorticoid
glucose
glutaraldehyde
　　g. cross-linked collagen
　　　(GAX)
glutathione
glycol
　　polyethylene g.
glycolate
glycopyrrolate
　　g. test
glycosaminoglycan
glycosaminoglycans
　　g. layer
　　g. uronate (GAGUA)
Glynazan
gold-198
Goldblatt
　　G. clamp
　　G. hypertension
　　G. phenomenon
GoLYTELY
　　G. solution
Gompertzian tumor kinetics
gonadal
　　g. differentiation
　　g. dysgenesis
gonadectomy
gonadoblastoma
gonadoliberin
gonadopathy
gonadotrophin
gonadotropin
　　human chorionic g.
　　　(HCG)
　　g. releasing hormone
gonangiectomy
gonecystolith
gonorrhoeae
　　Neisseria g.
Goodwin-Scott technique

Gore-Tex
gorget
  probe g.
Gorlin basal cell nevus
syndrome
goserelin
  g. acetate
Goulding procedure
Gouley's catheter
Grabstald (Memorial) staging
system
gracilis
  g. muscle
  g. myocutaneous
    neovagina
grade
  Gleason g.
  Gleason cancer g.
gradient-recalled acquisition in
  a steady state (GRASS)
grading
  histologic g.
  tumor g.
graft
  g. bed
  branched vascular g.
  buccal mucosal g.
  bypass g.
  Dacron g.
  loop forearm g.
  mucosal g.
  omental pedicle flap g.
  patch g.
  g. placement

prosthetic arterial g.
  g. spatulation
  split thickness skin g.
  synthetic vascular g.
  tube g.
granulocyte
granuloma
  g. inguinale
granulomatous prostatitis
granulosa cell tumor
grasper
  Allis tooth g.
  atraumatic g.
  traumatic locking g.
  umbilical port g.
grasping forceps
GRASS
  gradient-recalled acquisition
    in a steady state
gravel
Graves technique
gravity
  g.-dependent drainage
  specific g.
Grawitz' tumor
gray scale imaging
Greenfield filter
Greenwald
  G. Control Tip
    cystoscopic electrode
  G. needle
  G. sound
Gregoir-Lich procedure

NOTES

Greishaber self-retaining
    retractor
Grip-Tip suture guide
gross hematuria
Group
    Eastern Cooperative
        Oncology G. (ECOG)
growth
    g. factor beta
    g. regulation
guanadrel
guanethidine
    parenteral g.
guanoclor
guanoxan
guard-ring tocodynamometer
gubernacular vein
gubernaculum
Guerin
    valve of G.

guide
    catheter g.
    Grip-Tip suture g.
    Roth Grip-Tip suture g.
    suture g.
    g. wire
guide-eye instrument
guidewire
    Amplatz superstiff g.
    Bentson floppy-tipped g.
    Terumo g.
gumma
gun
    Bard Biopty g.
    biopsy g.
    Biopty g.
    Mentor g.
Guyon's sign
gynecomastia

H-600 Normothermic
Irrigating
habitus
   body h.
Haemophilus ducreyi
Halban procedure
Haldol
half-body irradiation
haloperidol
halothane
hamartoma
hammock
Handi-Cath catheter kit
haptoglobin
Harrington Deaver retractor
Harvard pump
harvester
   Arandel cell h
harvesting
Hashmat shunt
Hashmat-Waterhouse shunt
Hasson cannula
HCG
   human chorionic
     gonadotropin
healing
   wound h.
Heaney clamp
Heifitz clip
Heineke-Mikulicz principle
Heiss's loop
helical-ridged ureteral stent
helium-neon laser
Helmstein balloon
hemangioblastomatosis
   Von Hippel-Lindau
     cerebellar h.
hemangioma
   cavernous h.
hemangiopericytoma
hematocele
hematocelia

hematochyluria
hematocystis
hematocyturia
hematologic study
hematoma
   expanding
   retroperitoneal h.
   perirenal h.
   pulsatile h.
   renal h.
hematoporphyrin
hematospermatocele
hematospermia
hematoxylin
hematuresis
hematuria
   angioneurotic h.
   essential h.
   gross h.
   initial h.
   microscopic h.
   painful h.
   painless h.
   renal h.
   terminal h.
   total h.
   urethral h.
   vesical h.
hemiacidrin irrigation
hemihypertrophy
hemi-Kock
   h.-K. system
   h.-K. urinary diversion
heminephroureterectomy
hemipyonephrosis
hemiscrotectomy
hemoconcentration
hemocyanin
   keyhole limpet h.
   (KLH)
hemodialysis

Ham's F-10 Solution (for sperm)

hemodialyzer
    ultrafiltration h.
hemodynamics
hemofiltration
hemolytic uremic syndrome
hemonephrosis
hemophilia
    renal h.
hemopyelectasis,
   hemopyelectasia
hemorrhage
    renal h.
hemorrhagic nephritis
hemospermia
    h. spuria
    h. vera
hemostasis
hemostat
    curved h.
    ENDO-ASSIST
    disposable h.
hemuresis
Henoch-Schoelein purpura
heparin
    low-molecular weight h.
    (LMWH)
heparinization
heparinized saline
hepatic
    h. adhesion
    h. circulation
Hepatic-Aid
hepatitis
    h. A
    h. B
    h. C
hepatomegaly
hepatonephoric syndrome
hepatonephromegaly
hepatopathy
hepatorenal
    h. bypass
    h. syndrome
hepatosplenomegaly

hernia
    antevesical h.
    direct inguinal h.
    indirect inguinal h.
    inguinal h., direct
    inguinal h., indirect
    inguinal h.
    inguinoscrotal h.
    inguinosuperficial h.
    parastomal h.
    scrotal h.
    vesicle h.
hernia uteri inguinale
heroin
Herrick
    H. clamp
    H. kidney clamp
heterogeneity
    intratumor h.
hexamethonium
Heyer-Schulte stent
high
    h. frequency sonography
    h. lithotomy
    h. loop cutaneous
    ureterostomy
high-speed electrical tissue
  morcellator
hilar
    h. clamp
    h. structure scar tissue
Hinman
    H. procedure
    H. syndrome
hipran
hirsuitoid papilloma
hirsutism
    adrenal h.
histocompatibility
    h. complex
    h. testing
histologic grading
histology
histometry

histopathology
Histoplasma capsulatum
hitch
  psoas h.
HM4
  H. lithotriptor
HMB-45 monoclonal antibody
  marker
Hodgson technique of
  modified Lich procedure
holder
  Bovie h.
  Dale Foley catheter h.
  diamond jaw needle h.
  ENDO-ASSIST
    disposable needle h.
  Jacobson needle h.
  Mayo-Hegar needle h.
  microneedle h.
  microvascular needle h.
  needle h.
  Young needle h.
Holter
  vesicovaginal H.
Holyoke
  H. briefs
  H. pants
homatropine methylbromide
home
  h. care
  h. screening test
  h. uroflowmetry
hominis
  Mycoplasma h.

homogenous cooling
homovanillic acid (HVA)
honeymoon cystitis
hook
  h. electrode
  h. forceps
  nerve h.
  h. scissors
  h. tip laparoscopic
    electrode
  Whitaker h.
Hopkins telescope
hormonal
  h. downstaging
  h. therapy
hormone
  adrenal corticotropic h.
    (ACTH)
  h. antagonist
  follicle-stimulating h.
    (FSH)
  gonadotropin
    releasing h.
  LH-FSH releasing h.
  luteinizing hormone-
    releasing h. (LHRH)
Horner syndrome
horseshoe kidney
hospice care
hostility score
Hounsfield unit
Howard test
HPV
  human papillomavirus

NOTES

Huggins operation
Hulka clip
human
  h. chorionic
    gonadotropin (HCG)
  h. erectile dysfunction
  h. lyophilized dura
    cystoplasty
  h. papillomavirus (HPV)
  h. recombinant
    erythropoietin
Hunner
  H. stricture
  H. ulcer
HVA
  homovanillic acid
hyaluronic acid
hybridization
  Southern blot h.
Hybritech assay
hydatid cyst
hydatidocele
Hydergine
hydralazine
hydrobromide
hydrocalycosis
hydrocele
  abdominoscrotal h.
  congenital h.
  Dupuytren's h.
  h. feminae
  filarial h.
  funicular h.
  h. muliebris
  Nuck's h.
  postoperative h.
hydrocelectomy
hydrochloride
  bupivacaine h.
  ciprofloxacin h.
  lomefloxacin h.
  papaverine h.
  phenazopyridine h.
  procaine h.

  tolazoline h.
  yohimbine h.
hydrocirsocele
hydrocolpos
hydrocortisone
hydrodistention
Hydroflex penile prosthesis
hydrometrocolpos
hydromorphone
Hydromox
Hydromox-R
hydronephrosis
  bilateral h.
hydronephrotic
hydrophone
  Imotec needle h.
Hydro Plus coated guide wire
Hydropres-25
Hydropres-50
hydrorchis
hydroureter
hydroureteronephrosis
hydroxyapatite
hydroxyquinoline
hydroxystilbamidine
hydroxyurea
hydroxyzine
hydruria
hydruric
hymenoplasty
hymenotomy
hyoscyamine
  h. sulfate
hyperactivity
  detrusor h.
hyperaldosteronism
hypercalcemia
hypercalciuria
hypercarbia
hyperchloremic
  h. acidosis
  h. metabolic acidosis
hypercoagulability
hyperechoic

hyperfiltration
hyperhidrosis
hypermobility
  urethral h.
hypernatremia
hypernephroma
hyperorchidism
hyperosmolar perfusate
hyperoxaluria
hyperoxaluric stone
hyperparathyroidism
hyperperfusion
hyperplasia
  adrenal h.
  benign prostatic h.
  (BPH)
  bilobar h.
  congenital adrenal h.
  (CAH)
  fibromuscular h.
  nodular h. of prostate
  prostatic h.
  trilobar h.
hyperplastic nodule
hyperprolactinemia
hyperreflexia
  detrusor h.
hypersensitivity
hypertension
  allograft-mediated h.
  Goldblatt h.
  lithotripsy-induced h.
  renal h.
  renovascular h.

hyperthermia
  microwave h.
  transrectal prostatic h.
  (TPH)
hyperthyroidism
hypertrophy
  benign prostatic h.
  (BPH)
  bilobar h.
  compensatory
  testicular h.
  prostatic h.
  trilobar h.
hyperuricosuria
hypervolemia
hypnosis
hypoalbuminemia
hypocalcemia
hypoechoic
  h. cancer
hypoestrogenic urethritis
hypoestrogenism
hypogastric artery
hypokalemia
hypokalemic nephropathy
hyponatremia
hypophysectomy
hypoplasia
hypoplastic
  h. blind-ending
    spermatic vessels
  h. lung
hypospadiac

NOTES

hypospadias
  balanic h.
  penoscrotal h.
  perineal h.
hypotension
hypothermia
  renal h.
hypothermic
  h. effect

  h. perfusion
  h. storage
hypothyroidism
hypotonic bladder
hypovolemic shock
hypoxanthine
hypoxia
hysterocystopexy
hysteroscopy

iatrogenic
    i. trauma
ice
    i. cooling
    i. slush
    soft i.
idiopathic
    i. fibrous retroperitonitis
    i. retroperitoneal fibrosis
    i. sensory urgency
idiopathic sensory urgency
ifosfamide
IgA nephropathy
Iglesias
    I. fiberoptic resectoscope
    I. resectoscope
IgM nephropathy
ileal
    i. bladder
    i. conduit
    i. conduit urinary
      diversion
    i. interposition
    i. loop
    i. nipple valve
    i. reservoir
    i. sleeve
ileocecal
    i. bladder
    i. continent urinary
      reservoir
    i. reservoir
    i. segment
ileocecocystoplasty
    i. bladder augmentation
ileocolic urinary diversion
ileocolonic
    i. bladder
    i. neobladder
    i. pouch
    i. pouch urinary
      diversion

ileocolostomy
ileocystoplasty
ileosigmoid fistula
ileostomy
    i. rod
    Turnbull end-loop i.
ileoureteric stenosis
ileovesical fistula
ileus
    paralytic i.
iliac
iliorenal bypass
image
    axial i.
    i. cytometry
    i. processing
    sagittal i.
imaging
    B-mode i.
    gray scale i.
    LaparoScan laparoscopic
      ultrasonic i.
    magnetic resonance i.
      (MRI)
    radionuclide i.
    radionuclide renal i.
    sonoelasticity i.
imidazolecarboxamide
imipramine
immersion cooling
immortalization
immune suppression
immunoassay
    Abbott TDx monoclonal
      fluorescence
      polarization i.
immunobead-reacting antigen
immunocompromised
immunoenhancing
immunohistochemical detection
immunohistochemistry

immunoreactivity
   vasoactive intestinal
     polypeptide i. (VIP-IR)
immunosuppressive therapy
immunotherapy
Imotec needle hydrophone
impacted stone
Impact lithotriptor system
impactor
   electromechanical i.
     (EMI)
   stone i.
impassable ureter
implant
   penile i.
   Surgitek Flexi-Flate II
     penile i.
implantable penile venous
  compression device
implantation
   intracavitary i.
   radioactive seed i.
   real-time 3-D biplanar
     transperineal prostate i.
   ureter i.
impotence
   arteriogenic i.
   diabetic i.
   ejaculatory i.
   psychogenic i.
   vasculogenic i.
   venogenic i.
   venous leak i.
IMx PSA system
in
   i. situ
   i. vitro fertilization
   i. vivo
inadvertent enterotomy
Inapsine
incarceration
   penile i.
incidence
incidental adenoma

incision
   apron skin i.
   bilateral i.
   bilateral subcostal i.
   bilateral
     transabdominal i.
   Cherney i.
   chevron i.
   dorsal lumbotomy i.
   eleventh rib flank i.
   eleventh rib
     transperitoneal i.
   extended left
     subcostal i.
   flank i.
   Gibson i.
   Gibson-type i.
   lower abdominal
     transverse i.
   Mallard i.
   midline i.
   midline lower
     abdominal i.
   midline upper
     abdominal i.
   modified Gibson i.
   paramedian i.
   perineal i.
   Pfannenstiel i.
   posterior transthoracic i.
   stepladder i. technique
   subcostal flank i.
   subcostal
     transperitoneal i.
   surgical i.
   thoracoabdominal i.
   transpubic i.
   transverse i.
   transverse semilunar
     skin i.
   unilateral subcostal i.
   vertical midline i.
   xiphoid to pubis
     midline abdominal i.

inclusion cyst
incomplete duplication
incontinence
    anatomic stress i.
    overflow i.
    paradoxical i.
    passive i.
    post-prostatectomy i.
    reflex i.
    Resident Assessment
    Protocol for i.
    secondary i.
    stress i.
    stress urinary i.
    type III i.
    urge i., urgency i.
    urinary i.
    urinary exertional i.
    urinary stress i.
Inderal
index
    American Urological
    Association symptom i.
    (AUA symptom index)
    AUA symptom i.
    American Urological
    Association symptom
    index
    detrusor activity i.
    Karnofsky i.
    Maine Medical
    Assessment Program i.
    (MMAP index)
    i. of malnutrition

    mitosis-karyorrhexis i.
    (MKI)
    mitotic i.
    MMAP i.
    Maine Medical
    Assessment Program
    index
    obstruction i.
    penile-brachial i.
    p_2 penile brachial i.
    PSA i.
    symptom i.
    Uroflow i.
Indiana
    I. continent reservoir
    I. pouch
Indiana continent reservoir
    urinary diversion
indication
indigo
    i. calculus
    i. carmine
indigo-carmine-stained normal
    saline
indirect
    i. inguinal hernia
indolalkylamine alkaloid
induced
inducer
    interferon i.
indwelling
    i. catheter
infantile polycystic disease
    (IPCD)

NOTES

infarct
  Brewer's i.'s
  uric acid i.
infection
  fungal i.
  nosocomial i.
  nosocomial fungal i.
  urinary tract i. (UTI)
  wound i.
inferior rectal nerve
infertility
infiltration
  cellular i.
inflammation
  traumatic i.
inflammatory
  i. bowel disease
  i. renal mass
infradiaphragmatic
infrahepatic
infrared spectroscopy
infravesical
  i. prostatic obstruction
infundibulum
  caliceal i.
infusion pump
inguinal
  i. hernia
  i. reservoir inserter
inguinale
  granuloma i.
inguinoscrotal
  i. hernia
inguinosuperficial hernia
inhibin
inhibition
  antisense DNA i.
  bladder i.
inhibitor
  cyclooxygenase i.
  protease i.
initial hematuria
injection
  moxisylyte i.

  polytetrafluorethylene
    paste i.
  submucosal Teflon i.
injury
  renal vascular i.
  reperfusion i.
  vascular i.
inlay
  Turner-Warwick i.
inlet port
Inmed whistle tip urethral catheter
Innova home therapy system
Innova system
inserter
  Furlow cylinder i.
  inguinal reservoir i.
insipidus
  diabetes i.
instability
  detrusor i.
instrument
  Bard Biopty i.
  biopsy i.
  BIP biopsy i.
  DaVinci handle i.
  Dilamezinsert i.
  GIA i.
  guide-eye i.
  TA i.
instrumentation
  Karl Storz i.
  Microvasive i.
insufflation
insulated
  i. curved scissors
  i. straight scissors
insulin
insulin-like growth factor I
insult
  ischemic i.
intensified radiographic imaging system (IRIS)
interdigitating teeth

interferon
  i. inducer
  i. therapy
interferon type I
Intergroup Rhabdomyosarcoma
  Study (IRS)
interleukin
interleukin-2
intermittent catheterization
interna
  elastica i.
internal
  i. fiberoptic cable
  i. iliac artery
  i. pudendal artery
  i. pudendal vein
  i. urethrotomy
interposition
  ileal i.
interrupted suture
intersex condition
interstitial
  i. brachytherapy
  i. cell tumor of testis
  i. cystitis
  i. irradiation
intestinal
  i. fistula
  i. stricture
  i. surgery
  i. ureteral replacement
  i. ureter replacement
intimal fibroplasia
intracapsular dissection

intracavernosal injection
  treatment
intracavernous injection
  therapy
intracavitary implantation
intracavity implantation
intracellular flush effect
intracorporeal needle breakage
intractable
Intradop intraoperative
  Doppler
intralesional treatment
intralobar
intraluminal
  i. clot
  i. urethral pressure
intramural
  i. atheromatous disease
  i. ganglia
intraoperative mortality
intrapelvic filling defect
intraperitoneal adhesion
intraprostatic
  i. spiral
  i. stent
intrarenal
  i. collecting system
intratubular germ cell
  neoplasia (ITGCN)
intratumoral
intratumor heterogeneity
intraurethral pressure
intrauterine device
intravasation

NOTES

intravenous
  i. pyelogram (IVP)
  i. urogram
  i. urography
intravesical
  i. alum irrigation
  i. anastomosis
  i. migration
  i. pressure
  i. ureterolysis
intrinsic striated muscle of the urethra
introducer
  entrapment sack i.
  i. set
Intropin
intubated ureterotomy
intussusception
invasion
  vascular i.
Inversine
inverted testis
inverted V peritoneotomy
iodine-125
iodine hippurate scanning
Iodohippurate
Iodopyracet
iohexol
Ionamin
iontophoresis
IPCD
  infantile polycystic disease
iridium-192
IRIS
  intensified radiographic imaging system
irradiated tumor vaccine
irradiation
  i. failure
  half-body i.
  interstitial i.
  total body i. (TBI)
  ultraviolet i.

Irrigating
  H-600 Normothermic I.
irrigating fluid
irrigation
  continuous bladder i. (CBI)
  hemiacidrin i.
  intravesical alum i.
  rectum i.
  Renacidin i.
irrigator/aspirator
  Nezhat-Dorsey i.
irritable testis
irritative symptom
IRS
  Intergroup Rhabdomyosarcoma Study
ischemia
  myocardial i.
ischemic
  i. insult
ischiorectal abscess
island
  i. flap procedure
  i. pedicle flap
Ismelin
Isocal
isocarboxazid
isoflurane
isoniazid
isopropamide
isotope
  99mTc-MAG-3 i.
  99m technetium mercaptoacetythiglycine i.
  i. renography
isotropic scan
isoxsuprine
isradipine
Isuprel
ITGCN
  intratubular germ cell neoplasia

IVP   **IVU**
    intravenous pyelogram

J
    J. hook tip laparoscopic
      electrode
    J. wire
Jackson-Pratt drain
Jacobson needle holder
Janus System III
jaundice
jejunostomy
    needle-catheter j.
jelly
    Xylocaine j.
jet stream phenomenon
jeweler's forceps

Jewett sound
J-Maxx stent
Johnston
    J. buttonhole procedure
    J. procedure
Jonas penile prosthesis
Jones-Politano technique
J-pexy
    omental J.-p.
junction
    gap j.
junctional cyst
juxta-anal colostomy
juxtaglomerular

Kallman syndrome
Kaplan-Anderson Quality of
   Well-Being Scale
Kaplan-Meier curves
Kaposi's sarcoma
Karl
   K. Storz instrumentation
   K. Storz Lutzeyer
      lithotriptor
Karnofsky
   K. index
   K. performance status
      scale
   K. scale
karyometry
Kayexalate
KCL
Keeler panoramic loupe
Keflex
Kegel pelvic muscle exercise
Keith needle
Kelami classification
Kelly
   K. clamp
   K. operation
   K. plication
Kelly-Kennedy modification
Kemadrin
Kerlix
   K. wrap
Kessler-Kleinert suture
ketoconazole
ketorolac tromethamine
ketosteroid
keyhole limpet hemocyanin
   (KLH)
Keystone technique
Khafagy modified ileocecal
   cystoplasty urinary diversion
kidney
   k. allograft

artificial k.
Ask-Upmark k.
cadaver k.
k. carbuncle
k. clearance
k. failure
k. function
horseshoe k.
medullary sponge k.
multicystic k. (MCK)
multicystic dysplastic k.
k. pedicle clamp
solitary k.
k. transplant
k. transplantation
kidney, ureter, bladder
   radiography (KUB
   radiography)
Kinesed
kinetics
   Bromodeoxyuridine
      cell k.
   Gompertzian tumor k.
kinking
"kissing" prostatic lobes
kit
   Pros-Check k.
Kleinert's
   K. pants
   K. Safe and Dry panty
      and pad system
KLH
   keyhole limpet hemocyanin
knife
   cold k.
   Collings k.
   Collings electrosurgery k.
   k. electrode
   endarterectomy k.
   optical laser k.
   Orandi k.

knot
    curved-needle
      surgeon's k.
    surgeon's k.
knot pusher
    Clarke-Reich k. p.
    Gazayerli k. p.
knotting
    stochastic k.
Kocher
    K. clamp
    K. maneuver
Kock
    K. nipple
    K. pouch
    K. pouch cutaneous
      urinary diversion
Kockogram

Kock's technique
Kollmann's dilator
Kossa stain
K-Phos
Krause arm rest
Krebs' solution
Kreha
    polysaccharide K. (PSK)
Kretz
    K. Combison
    Ultrasound Scanner
    K. ultrasound system
krypton laser
KTP\532 laser
KTP laser probe
KUB radiography
kyphoscoliosis

LAAL
lower anterior axillary line
labetalol
labia
l. major muscle
l. minor muscle
laceration
longitudinal l.
lower pole l.
rectal l.
vascular l.
lactate
Ringer's l.
lactate dehydrogenase
lactic
l. acid dehydrogenase (LDH)
l. dehydrogenase
lactulose
lacunar abscess
LAK cell
lymphokine-activated killer cell
Lalonde hook forceps
lamina
l. propria
laminectomy
LaparoScan laparoscopic ultrasonic imaging
laparoscopic
l. lymphocelectomy
l. needle driver
l. nephrectomy
l. pelvic lymphadenectomy
l. varicocelectomy
l. varix ligation
laparoscopy
laparotomy
l. pack
Laplace's law
LapSac

Larodopa
laser
alexandrite l.
argon l.
Candela Model MDL 2000 l.
CO_2 l.
Coherent Model 90-K l.
l. Doppler flowmeter
dye l.
helium-neon l.
krypton l.
KTP\532 l.
Lithognost l.
l. lithotripsy
l. lithotriptor
Nd:YAG l.
neodymium:yttrium garnet laser
neodymium:YAG l.
neodymium:yttrium garnet l. (Nd:YAG laser, Nd:YAG laser)
pulsed-dye neodymium:YAG l.
Q-switched alexandrite l.
l. surgery
l. therapy
l. tissue welding
l. tissue welding solder
tunable pulsed dye l.
ultrasound guided l.
YAG l.
laser-induced intracorporeal shock wave lithotripsy (LISL)
LaserMed laser pointer
Laserscope KTP\532
Laserscope YAG\1064
lasertripsy
Lasix

latency
    pudendal nerve terminal
      motor l.
lateral lithotomy
latex
    l. allergy
Latzko partial colpocleisis
lavage solution
law
    Laplace's l.
    Poiseuille's l.
    Weigert-Meyer l.
layer
    glycosaminoglycans l.
    submucosal vaginal
      smooth
      musculofascial l.
LDH
    lactic acid dehydrogenase
Le
    L. Bag
    L. Bag urinary diversion
    L. Fort sound
Leach technique
Leadbetter procedure
leakage
    postmicturition
    continuous l.
leak point pressure
leiomyoma
leiomyosarcoma
Lembert
    L. inverting
      seromuscular suture
    L. suture
length
    functional profile l.
lens
    120-degree l.
    30-degree l.
    70-degree l.
    objective l.
lesion
    acetowhite l.

    cauda equina l.
    dye sham intrarenal l.
    macroscopic l.
    metastatic l.
    papillary l.
    precancerous l.
    traumatic l.
    vascular l.
leucovorin
leukemia
leukocytosis
leukopenia
leukoplakia
leuprolide
    l. acetate
leuprolide acetate
Levamphetamine
Levarterenol
Levatol
levator ani muscle
Leveen syringe
levodopa
levorphanol
Levsinex
Levsin/SL
Lewis X antigen
Lewy syringe
Leydig
    L. cell adenoma
    L. cell tumor
LGV
    lymphogranuloma venereum
LH-FSH releasing hormone
LHRH
    luteinizing hormone-
    releasing hormone
libido
Librax
Lich
    L. extravesical technique
    L. procedure
    L. technique

Lich-Gregoir
  L.-G. anastomosis
  L.-G. ureterolysis
lidocaine
lienorenal ligament
life
  quality of l.
ligament
  lienorenal l.
  medial umbilical l.
  pubourethral l.'s
  sacrotuberous l.
ligation
  laparoscopic varix l.
ligature
  silk l.
  suture l.
light
  l. cable
  l. electrocautery
  l. microscopy
limb deformity
**limited obturator node
  dissection**
line
  anterior axillary l.
  (AAL)
  Brodel's l.
  lower anterior axillary l.
  (LAAL)
  lower midclavicular l.
  (LMCL)
  midclavicular l. (MCL)

  upper midclavicular l.
  (UMCL)
linear stapling device
Lingeman
  L. 3 in 1 procedure
  drape
  L. TUR drape
linsidomine chlorohydrate
lipogranulomatosis
lipoid nephrosis
lipoma
lipomeningocele
lipomyelomeningocele
lipopolysaccharide
liposarcoma
LISL
  laser-induced intracorporeal
  shock wave lithotripsy
lithagogue
lithectomy
lithiasis
  cystine l.
  uric acid l.
Lithoclast
  L. lithotriptor
  Swiss L.
lithoclast
lithocystotomy
lithodialysis
Lithognost laser
litholabe
litholapaxy
litholysis
litholyte

NOTES

lithometer
lithomyl
lithonephritis
lithophone
lithoscope
Lithostar
    L. lithotriptor
    L. Plus
    Siemens L.
Lithostat
lithotome
lithotomist
lithotomy
    bilateral l.
    high l.
    lateral l.
    marian l.
    median l.
    perineal l.
    prerectal l.
    suprapubic l.
    vaginal l.
    vesical l.
lithotresis
    ultrasonic l.
lithotripsy
    electrohydraulic l.
    extracorporeal
      piezoelectric l. (EPL)
    extracorporeal shock
      wave l. (ESWL)
    laser l.
    laser-induced
      intracorporeal shock
      wave l. (LISL)
    piezoelectric l.
    pressure regulated
      electrohydraulic l.
    l. retreatment
    shock wave l.
    ultrasonic l.
lithotripsy-induced hypertension
lithotriptic

lithotriptor, lithotripter
    Breakstone l.
    Calcutript
    Electrohydraulic l.
    Calcutript
    electrohydraulic l.
    Circon-ACMI l.
    Direx Tripter X-1 l.
    Dornier HM3 l.
    Dornier HM4 l.
    EDAP LT.01 l.
    electrohydraulic l.
    extracorporeal shock
      wave l.
    HM4 l.
    Karl Storz Lutzeyer l.
    laser l.
    Lithoclast l.
    Lithostar l.
    Medstone STS l.
    MFL 5000 l.
    Northgate SD-3 dual-
      purpose l.
    percutaneous
      ultrasonic l.
    piezoelectric l.
    piezoelectric shock
      wave l.
    shock wave l.
    Siemens l.
    Sonotrode l.
    Wolf l.
    Wolf Piezolith l.
    Wolf Piezolith 2300 l.
    Wolf Sonolith l.
lithotriptoscope
lithotriptoscopy
lithotrite
    Marmite l.
lithotrity
lithuresis
lithureteria
LMCL
    lower midclavicular line

LMWH
> low-molecular weight
> heparin

lobes
> "kissing" prostatic l.

localization
> target l.

local scarring

location
> tumor l.

lomefloxacin
> l. hydrochloride
> l. TMP/SMX

longitudinal
> l. enterotomy
> l. laceration
> l. nephrotomy of Boyce
> l. subepithelial venous
> plexus

loop
> brain stem-sacral l.
> cerebral-sacral l.
> Davis l.
> l. forearm graft
> Heiss's l.
> ileal l.
> resectoscope l.
> l. stoma
> l. transverse colostomy
> vesical-sacral-sphincter l.

loop-o-gram
loop-tipped electrode
Lopressor

loupe
> Keeler panoramic l.
> surgical l.
> wide-angled l.

low-compliance bladder
lower
> l. abdominal transverse
> incision
> l. anterior axillary line
> (LAAL)
> l. midclavicular line
> (LMCL)
> l. pole laceration

low loop cutaneous
> ureterostomy

low-molecular weight heparin
> (LMWH)

Lowsley tractor
L-PAM
lubricant
> Surgilube l.

Lubri-flex ureteral stent
Lubriglide-coated guide wire
Luer-Lok connector
lues
lumbar nephrectomy
lumbosacral
> l. fascia
> l. trunk

lumen
Lunderquist wire
lung
> hypoplastic l.

Lupron Depot

NOTES

lupus nephritis
luteinizing hormone
luteinizing hormone-releasing
  hormone (LHRH)
lymph
  l. node metastasis
  l. scrotum
lymphadenectomy
  laparoscopic pelvic l.
  para-aortic l.
  pelvic l.
  prophylactic l.
  retroperitoneal l.
  thoracoabdominal
    retroperitoneal l.
lymphangiogram
lymphangiography
lymphangioma

lymphatic package
lymphedema
lymphocele
lymphocelectomy
  laparoscopic l.
lymphocyst
lymphocytes
  tumor infiltrating l.
    (TIL)
lymphogranuloma venereum
  (LGV)
lymphokine-activated
  l.-a. killer cell (LAK
    cell)
lymphoma
Lyon's ring-constrictive band
lysis

99m
99m technetium diethylenetriamine pentaacetic acid scan
99m technetium mercaptoacetythiglycine isotope

machine
Belzer m.
MOX TM-100 portable renal preservation m.
perfusion m.
portable renal preservation m.

Macrobid

macrocrystal

macrocyst
adrenocortical m.

Macrodantin

macromolecular uronate (MMUA)

macropenis

macrophallus

macroscopic lesion

Madsen-Iversen scoring system

MAG-3
mercaptotriglycylglycine

magnesium ammonium phosphate

magnesium oxide

magnetic
m. bore
m. resonance imaging (MRI)
m. resonance spectroscopy

MAGPI
meatal advancement and glansplasty

Maine Medical Assessment Program index (MMAP index)

Mainz
M. pouch
M. pouch cutaneous urinary diversion
M. pouch II

malacoplakia

malakoplakia

male catheter

Malecot
M. catheter
M. reentry catheter

malemission

malformation
arteriovenous m.
cloacal m.

malignant renal mass

Mallard incision

malleable
m. blade
m. retractor

malnutrition
index of m.

malrotation

maltose tetrapalmitate

mammalgia

mAMSA
amsacrine

maneuver
Crede m.
Fowler-Stephens m.
Kocher m.
Valsalva m.

manipulation
direct m.
postureteroscopic m.

mannitol

Mann-Whitney test

manometer

Mansson operation

Mantel-Haenszel test

Marcaine

marcescens
  Serratia m.
margin
  dissection m.
marian lithotomy
Marion's disease
marker
  biochemical m.
  biological m.
  HMB-45 monoclonal
    antibody m.
  molecular m.
  tumor m.
  tumor cell m.
Marmite lithotrite
Marshall-Marchetti-Krantz
  M.-M.-K. operation
  M.-M.-K. procedure
  M.-M.-K. urethropexy
Marshall-Marchetti test
marsupialization
Martius flap
mass
  asymptomatic m.
  congenital renal m.
  cystic m.
  extrarenal m.
  flank m.
  inflammatory renal m.
  malignant renal m.
  neoplastic renal m.
  renal m.
  traumatic renal m.
  tubular excretory m.
  vascular renal m.
massage
  prostatic m.
masturbation
  traumatic m.
material
  suture m.
Mathieu-Horton-Devine flip-
  flap
Mathieu procedure

matrix calculus
mattress suture
maturation
Mavigraph color video printer
Maxaquin
maximum
  m. bladder capacity
  m. cystometric capacity
Maydl procedure
Mayer-Rokitansky syndrome
Mayo
  M. scissors
  M. stand
Mayo-Hegar needle holder
Mazicon
mazindol
Mazzariello-Caprini forceps
McBurney retractor
McCall culdoplasty
McCrea sound
McGaw's plastic bottle
MCK
  multicystic kidney
MCL
  midclavicular line
  MCL port
McNemar test
MCV
  molluscum contagiosum
  virus
MEA-I
  multiple endocrine
  adenomatosis type I
MEA-II
  multiple endocrine
  adenomatosis type II
Meares-Stamey technique
measurement
  RigiScan m.
  urethral pressure m.
measurements
  voiding urethral
  pressure m. (VUPP)

meatal
   m. advancement
   m. advancement and
   glansplasty (MAGPI)
   m. spreader
meatal spreader
meatoplasty
   V-flap m.
meatorrhaphy
meatoscope
meatoscopy
meatotome
meatotomy
   m. scissors
   ureteral m.
meatus
mecamylamine
mechanism
   Albarran m.
   Mitrofanoff m.
Mecholyl
meconium peritonitis
Medena tube
medial
   m. fibroplasia
   m. umbilical ligament
median
   m. bar formation
   m. bar of Mercier
   m. lithotomy
mediastinal tumor
medical evaluation
Medihistory

medium
   contrast m.
medroxyprogesterone
   m. acetate
Medstone
   M. IRIS system
   M. STS lithotripsy
   system
   M. STS lithotriptor
Medtrax Urology Database
Medtrax Urology software
medullary
   m. oxygenation
   m. sponge kidney
   m. thyroid carcinoma
medulloblastoma
megabladder
Megace
megacystic syndrome
megacystis
megacystis-megaureter
   m.-m. association
   m.-m. syndrome
megalopenis
megalophallus
megaloureter
megalourethra
megaureter
   primary obstructive m.
megaurethra
megestrol acetate
meglumine diatrizoate
melanoma

NOTES

melanotic neuroectodermal
tumor of infancy
mellitus
  diabetes m.
melphalan
membrane
  m. catheter technique
  cloacal m.
  m. current
meningomyelocele
menouria
MENS
  multiple endocrine
  neoplasia syndrome
Mentor
  M. gun
  M. inflatable penile
  prosthesis
  M. IPP prosthesis
  M. Response VCD
Mentor-Alpha I penile
  prosthesis
Mentor-Piston VCD
Mentor-Touch VCD
mepenzolate
meperidine
mephentermine
mercaptotriglycylglycine
  (MAG-3)
Mercier's bar
Mersilene
  M. strut
  M. suture
mesangial proliferative
  glomerulonephritis
mesenteric
mesenterorenal bypass
mesoblastic nephroma
mesometrium
mesonephric duct
mesoridazine
mesothelioma
  benign m. of genital
  tract

Mestinon
metabolic
  m. evaluation
  m. range
  m. rate
  m. stone disease
metabolism
  protein m.
  tryptophan m.
metaiodobenzylguanidine
  (MIBG)
metal
  m. bar retractor
  m. clip
metallic staple
metalloproteinase
metallothionein
metal-tipped stent pusher
metanephrine
metaplasia
  myeloid m.
metaraminol
metastasis
  brain m.
  lymph node m.
  neoplasm m.
metastatic
  m. dissemination
  m. lesion
  m. prostatic carcinoma
  m. renal cell carcinoma
  (MRCC)
Metatensin
metaxalone
meter
  Aleo m. S-D2
methacholine
methadone
methamphetamine
methantheline
methapyrilene
methdilazine
Methedrine
Methiodal

methixene
method
   Metzer-Boyce m.
   triangulation m.
   triangulation stapling m.
methotrexate
methotrexate, vinblastine,
   Adriamycin, and cisplatin
   (MVAC)
methoxyphenamine
methscopolamine bromide
methylatropine nitrate
methylbromide
   homatropine m.
methyl CCNU
methyldopa
   parenteral m.
methyldopate
methylene blue
methylnitrate
   atropine m.
methylphenidate
methylprednisolone
   m. acetate
methyltestosterone
methysergide
metoclopramide
metoprolol
MetroGel
metronidazole
metyrapone
   m. stimulation test
Metzenbaum scissors
Metzer-Boyce method

MFL 5000 lithotriptor
Miami pouch
MIBG
   metaiodobenzylguanidine
Michaelis-Gutmann bodies
Michal
   M. II procedure
   M. I procedure
microcystic disease of renal
   medulla
microimplant
microlith
microlithiasis
microneedle holder
micropenis
microphallus
microscopic hematuria
microscopy
   electron m.
   light m.
   polarization m.
   scanning electron m.
   (SEM)
microsphere
   Super-Bright m.
Microspike
   M. approximator clamp
microsurgical inguinal
   varicocelectomy
microtransducer technique
microvascular
   m. clamp
   m. needle holder

NOTES

Microvasive
    M. instrumentation
    M. stent
Microvasive ASAP 18
microwave hyperthermia
micturating cystogram
micturition
    m. cystourethrography
midazolam
midclavicular line (MCL)
midline
    m. incision
    m. lower abdominal
      incision
    m. upper abdominal
      incision
midureteral calculus
migration
    calculus m.
    intravesical m.
milk-alkali syndrome
Millar catheter
"Millie" female urinal
Millin
    M. bladder retractor
    M. forceps
mind-bladder syndrome
mineralocorticoid
minilaparotomy
minimal-change
    m.-c. disease
    m.-c. nephrotic
      syndrome
mini-VAB
    vinblastine, actinomycin-D,
      and bleomycin
minoxidil
Mission VED VCD
Misstique female external
  urinary collector
mitomycin, mitomycin C
mitosis-karyorrhexis index
  (MKI)
mitotic index

Mitrofanoff
    M. conduit
    M. mechanism
    M. principle
    M. stoma
    M. technique
    M. valve
mitrogenic effect
MK-906
MKI
    mitosis-karyorrhexis index
MMAP index
MMUA
    macromolecular uronate
Moban
mobilization
Mobin-Uddin umbrella
model
Moderil
modification
    Kelly-Kennedy m.
    Muzsnai m.
    Raz m.
modified
    m. Essed-Schroeder
      corporoplasty
    m. Gibson incision
modulation
    obstruction-induced m.
    pressure amplitude m.
mogen clamp
Moh's microsurgery technique
mold
molecular
    m. cloning
    m. genetic alteration
    m. marker
    m. study
molindone
molluscum contagiosum virus
  (MCV)
Monfort operation
monitoring
    ambulatory m.

ambulatory
  urodynamic m.
fluoroscopic m.
nocturnal penile
  tumescence m.
NPT m.
Monitur
monoclonal antibody
Monocryl suture
Monodox
Monodral
monofilament suture
monohydrate
  doxycycline m.
monotherapy
Moraxella
morbidity
  febrile m.
  operative m.
  treatment m.
morcellator
  Cook tissue m.
  electric tissue m.
  high-speed electrical
    tissue m.
  tissue m.
morphine
morphometric criteria
morphometry
mortality
  intraoperative m.
  m. rate
mosaicism
  XX male m.

Moschcowitz procedure
motility
motor
  m. syringe
  m. urgency
movable testis
movement
  pelvic floor m.
moxisylyte injection
MOX TM-100 portable renal
  preservation machine
Moynihan clamp
MRCC
  metastatic renal cell
  carcinoma
MRI
  magnetic resonance imaging
mucosal graft
mucosa-to-mucosa anastomosis
mucositis
mulberry calculus
müllerian
  m. duct
  m. duct cyst
  m. inhibiting factor
  m. remnants
multicystic
  m. dysplastic kidney
  m. kidney (MCK)
multifiber catheter
multifire clip applicator
multiloaded clip applier
multiload occlusive clip
  applicator

NOTES

multilocular
  m. cyst
  m. cystic nephroma
multiple
  m. endocrine
    adenomatosis type I
    (MEA-I)
  m. endocrine
    adenomatosis type II
    (MEA-II)
  m. endocrine neoplasia
    syndrome (MENS)
  m. recurrent renal colic
  m. stages
mural thrombus
muscle
  adductor brevis m.
  adductor longus m.
  dartos m.
  external anal
    sphincter m.
  gracilis m.
  labia major m.
  labia minor m.
  levator ani m.
  obturator internus m.
  periurethral striated m.
  psoas m.
  pubococcygeus m.
  rectourethral m.
  submucosal vaginal m.
  superficial trigonal m.
  urogenital sphincter m.

muscularis tunnel closure
musculocutaneous
mushroom catheter
mutation
Muzsnai modification
MVAC
  methotrexate, vinblastine,
    Adriamycin, and cisplatin
myasthenia
mycobacteria
Mycobacterium bovis
Mycoplasma
  M. hominis
mycoplasma urethritis
Mycotrim triphasic culture
  system
myelodysplasia
myelography
myeloid metaplasia
myelolipoma
myeloma
myelomeningocele
myelosuppression
myocardial
  m. ischemia
  m. revascularization
myoclonus-opsoclonus
  syndrome
myocutaneous flap
MyoTrac EMG
Mytelase

N

**N-acetyl-β-glucosaminidase
(NAG)**
nadolol
nafoxidine
NAG
   N-acetyl-β-glucosaminidase
nalidixic acid
naloxone hydrochloride
NANC inhibitory transmitter
   nonadrenergic
   noncholinergic inhibitory
   transmitter
naphazoline
naphthylamine
nappies
   electronic recording n.
narcotic
Nardil
National
   N. Prostatic Cancer
   Project
   N. Wilms' Tumor Study
   (NWTS-4)
natural killer cell
nausea
Navane
navicularis
   fossa n.
NBC
   nephroblastomatosis
   complex
NC
   nephrocalcin
Nd:YAG laser
   neodymium:yttrium garnet
   laser
necrosis
   tubular n.
necrotizing fasciitis
needle
   ASAP prostate biopsy n.
   n. biopsy

   Biopty cut n.
   blunt n.
   butterfly n.
   CE-24 n.
   circle n.
   concentric n.
   Corson n.
   cutting LR n.
   n. driver
   n. electrode
   electrosurgical n.
   Greenwald n.
   n. holder
   Keith n.
   Promex biopsy n.
   PS-2 n.
   n. tip laparoscopic
   electrode
   Tru-Cut biopsy n.
   TT-3 n.
   Veress n.
needle-catheter
   n.-c. jejunostomy
Neisseria gonorrhoeae
Neisser's syringe
Nembutal
neoadjuvant
   n. antiandrogenic
   treatment
   n. hormonal deprivation
neobladder
   decompensated n.
   gastric n.
   ileocolonic n.
neocystostomy
neodymium:YAG laser
neodymium:YAG laser therapy
**neodymium:yttrium garnet
   laser (Nd:YAG laser,
   Nd:YAG laser)**
neointimal
Neoloid

neomycin
neoplasia
    cervical intraepithelial n.
    (CIN)
    intratubular germ cell n.
    (ITGCN)
    prostatic
    intraepithelial n. (PIN)
neoplasm
    bladder n.
    genitourinary n.
    n. metastasis
    prostatic n.
    retroperitoneal n.
    n. staging
neoplastic
    n. renal mass
    n. transformation
neostigmine
neourethra
Neo-Vadrin
neovagina
    gracilis myocutaneous n.
    skin graft n.
neovascular bundle
nephradenoma
nephralgia
nephralgic
nephrasthenia
nephratonia, nephratony
nephrectasis, nephrectasia
nephrectomy
    abdominal n.
    adjuvant n.
    anterior n.
    apical polar n.
    Balkan n.
    extracorporeal partial n.
    laparoscopic n.
    lumbar n.
    paraperitoneal n.
    partial n.
    posterior n.

    radical n.
    transplant n.
nephredema
nephrelcosis
nephritic
    n. calculus
    n. syndrome
nephritis, pl. nephritides
    acute n.
    acute focal bacterial n.
    (AFBN)
    acute interstitial n.
    hemorrhagic n.
    lupus n.
    salt-losing n.
    serum n.
    suppurative n.
    trench n.
nephroblastoma
nephroblastomatosis
    n. complex (NBC)
nephrocalcin (NC)
nephrocalcinosis
nephrocapsectomy
nephrocele
nephrocelom
nephrogenetic, nephrogenic
nephrogenous
nephrogram
nephrography
nephrohydrosis
nephrolith
nephrolithiasis
    calcium oxalate n.
nephrolithotomy
    anatrophic n.
    percutaneous n. (PCNL)
    simultaneous bilateral
    percutaneous n. (SBPN)
nephrology
nephrolysin
nephrolysis
nephrolytic

nephroma
    cystic n.
    mesoblastic n.
    multilocular cystic n.
nephron-sparing surgery
nephropathy
    analgesic n.
    Balkan n.
    Danubian endemic
    familial n.
    hypokalemic n.
    IgA n.
    IgM n.
nephropexy
nephrophthisis
    familial juvenile n.
nephroptosis, nephroptosia
nephropyelitis
nephropyeloplasty
nephropyosis
nephrorrhaphy
nephrosclerosis
nephroscope
    flexible n.
    rigid n.
    n. sheath
    Storz n.
    Wolf percutaneous
    universal n.
nephroscopy
    anatrophic n.
    flexible n.
nephrosis
    acute n.

    amyloid n.
    familial n.
    lipoid n.
nephrospasia, nephrospasis
nephrostogram
nephrostolithotomy
nephrostomy
    n. catheter
    percutaneous n.
    n. tube
nephrotic
nephrotomic cavity
nephrotomogram
nephrotomography
nephrotomy
    anatrophic n.
    n. tube
nephrotoxic
nephrotoxicity
nephrotoxin
nephrotrophic
nephrotropic
nephrotuberculosis
nephroureterectomy
    radical n.
nephroureterocystectomy
nephroureteroscopy
nerve
    n. block
    dorsal n. of penis
    genitofemoral n.
    n. hook
    inferior rectal n.

NOTES

nerve *(continued)*
    perineal n.
    pudendal n.
nerve-sparing
    n.-s. radical
        prostatectomy
nervous bladder
Nesbit
    N. plication
    N. procedure
neuraminidase
neuroblastoma
neurofibroma
neurofibromatosis
    Von Recklinghausen's n.
neurogenic bladder
neuron-specific enolase (NSE)
neuropathic
    n. bladder
    n. dysfunction
neuropharmacology
neurophysiology
neurosis
    bladder n.
neurotrophin
neuroureterectomy
Neutra-Phos
Neutra-Phos-K
neutron
neutropenia
Nezhat-Dorsey
    irrigator/aspirator
nialamide
Nichol's bowel preparation
nifedipine
nil disease
nilutamide
nimodipine
nipple
    Kock n.
    n. valve
nitrate
    methylatropine n.
nitric oxide

4-nitrobiphenyl
nitrofurantoin
nitrofurantoin monohydrate
nitrofurazone
nitroglycerin
nitroprusside
nitrosamine
nitrosourea
nitrous oxide
N-myc oncogene
N-nitrosamine
nocturia
nocturnal
    n. enuresis
    n. penile tumescence
        (NPT)
    n. penile tumescence
        monitoring
    n. tumescence
    n. tumescence self-
        monitoring
node distribution
nodosa
    polyarteritis n.
nodular hyperplasia of
    prostate
nodule
    hyperplastic n.
nomogram
nonadrenergic noncholinergic
    inhibitory transmitter
    (NANC inhibitory
    transmitter)
nonbacterial prostatitis
noncommunicating diverticulum
noncrushing bowel clamp
nondilating reflux
nondismembered anastomosis
nonfusion
non-germ cell carcinoma
nongonococcal urethritis
noninvasive
    n. diagnosis
    n. tumor

nonkeratinizing squamous
epithelium
nonseminomatous
  n. testicular carcinoma
  n. tumor
nonsteroidal
  n. anti-inflammatory
    drug (NSAID)
norepinephrine
Norflex
norfloxacin
normal
  n. detrusor contractility
  n. saline solution
Normodyne
normospermatogenic sterility
normothermic effect
Norpramin
Northgate SD-3 dual-purpose
  lithotriptor
nortriptyline
no-scalpel vasectomy
nosocomial
  n. fungal infection
  n. infection
Nottingham ureteral dilator
novo
  de n.

NPT
  nocturnal penile tumescence
  NPT monitoring
NSAID
  nonsteroidal anti-
  inflammatory drug
NSE
  neuron-specific enolase
NTZ Long-acting
Nuck's hydrocele
nuclear
  n. isotope scan
  n. matrix alteration
  n. roundness factor
nuclear isotope scan
number
  shock n.
nutrition
  enteral n.
  parenteral n.
  perioperative n.
  total parenteral n.
NWTS-4
  National Wilms' Tumor
  Study
nycturia
nylidrin
nystatin

NOTES

oat cell
obesity
objective lens
oblique obturator
obliterans
    balanitis xerotica o.
    (BXO)
obliteration of psoas shadow
obstructed
    o. pelvis
    o. testis
obstruction
    bladder outflow o.
    bladder outlet o.
    bowel o.
    ejaculatory duct o.
    o. index
    infravesical prostatic o.
    outlet o.
    ureteral o.
    ureteropelvic o.
    ureteropelvic junction o.
    ureterovesical o.
    urethral o.
obstruction-induced modulation
obstructive uropathy
obturator
    blunt-tipped o.
    o. internus muscle
    o. lymphatic chain
    oblique o.
    Timberlake o.
occlusion
    balloon o.
    balloon ureteral o.
    tourniquet o.
    urethral o.
occlusive clamp
occult bleeding
Ochoa syndrome
O'Conor drape
offset lens ureteroscope

ofloxacin
OK-432
OKT3 anti-T-cell antibody
oligoasthenoteratozoospermia
oligohydramnios
    o. complex
oligospermia, oligospermatism
oligozoospermatism,
   oligozoospermia
oliguresia, oliguresis
oliguria
olive-tipped catheter
Olympus
    O. continuous flow
    resectoscope
    O. OTV-S2 miniature
    camera
    O. video urology
    procedure system
Ombrédanne operation
omental
    o. J-pexy
    o. pedicle flap graft
omentum
omeprazole
Omniphase penile prosthesis
oncocytoma
oncogene
    N-myc o.
oncogene-induced
   carcinogenesis
oncologist
oncology
ondansetron
one-hour office pad test
oneirogmus
one-stage
    o.-s. procedure
    o.-s. repair
onlay
    o. island flap

onlay *(continued)*
   o. island flap
    urethroplasty
opacification
opacify
open pyelotomy
operation *(See also* procedure, repair)
   Bassini o.
   Bozeman o.
   Bricker o.
   Brunschwig o.
   Crespo o.
   Foley o.
   Furlow-Fisher modification of Virag 1 o.
   Gil-Vernet o.
   Huggins o.
   Kelly o.
   Mansson o.
   Marshall-Marchetti-Krantz o.
   Monfort o.
   Ombrédanne o.
   Rovsing o.
   Smith-Boyce o.
   Torek o.
   Virag o.
   Wheelhouse o.
operative
   o. morbidity
   o. staging
opiate
opioid
optical laser knife
optics
   fiber o.
Optilume prostate balloon dilator
optimum cooling range
Orandi knife
orchectomy
orchialgia

orchiatrophy
orchichorea
orchidalgia
orchidectomy
orchiditis
orchidometer
   Prader o.
   Test-Size o.
orchidopexy
orchidoptosis
orchidorraphy
orchiectomy
   radical inguinal o.
orchiepididymitis
orchilytic
orchiocele
orchiodynia
orchioneuralgia
orchiopathy
orchiopexy
   Fowler-Stephens o.
   transseptal o.
orchioplasty
orchiorrhaphy
orchiotherapy
orchiotomy
orchitic
orchitis
   o. parotidea
   traumatic o.
   o. variolosa
orchotomy
Oreticyl
organ
   artificial o.
   o. donation
orifice
   bell-shaped o.
   epispadiac o.
   sharp-edged o.
   ureteral o.
Ormond's disease
orphenadrine
Orthopara-DDD

orthotopic bladder
orthovoltage teletherapy
Orthoxine
Osbon ErecAid VCD
oscheitis
oschelephantiasis
oscheohydrocele
oscheoplasty
osmolarity
ossification
osteitis
osteogenic sarcoma
osteosarcoma
osteotomy
ostial atherosclerotic plaque
ostium
ostomy
Otis urethrotome
Otrivin
outcome and process
    assessment
outlet
    bladder o.
    o. obstruction
ovarian carcinoma
ovarii
    tunica albuginea o.

over-and-over suture
overdistension
overdosing
overflow incontinence
overload
    volume o.
oxalate
    calcium o.
    o. calculus
oxaluria
    calcium o.
oxidase
    xanthine o.
oxide
    nitric o.
oxybutynin
    o. chloride
Oxycel
oxychlorosene sodium
oxycodone
oxygenation
    medullary o.
oxymorphone
oxyphencyclimine

NOTES

P4
> BioGel P.

pacemaker
> pervenous p.

pack
> laparotomy p.

package
> lymphatic p.

packing forceps
Pacquin ureterolysis
padding
> Spenco p.

Padgett dermatome
pads
> Active Living
> incontinence p.
> Sani Pads medicated
> cleansing p.

Paget's disease
Pagitane
pain
> p. assessment
> p. control

painful hematuria
painless hematuria
PALA
palladium-103
palliative
> p. care

pallidum
> *Treponema p.*

Palmaz
> P. balloon-expandable
> stent
> P. stent

palpation
palsy
> cerebral p.

Pamine
p-amino-hippuric acid
pampinocele
pancreas

pancreatectomy
pancreatic carcinoma
pancreaticocystostomy
pancreatitis
panendoscope
pants
> Ashton p.
> Dignity incontinence p.
> Holyoke p.
> Kleinert's p.
> Suretys p.
> Ultrafem p.

PAP
> prostatic acid phosphatase

papaverine
> p. hydrochloride

papillary lesion
papilloma
> hirsuitoid p.

papillomatosis coronae
papillomavirus
> human p. (HPV)

Pap-Kaps
papulosis
> bowenoid p.

para-aortic lymphadenectomy
paradoxical incontinence
paralytic ileus
paramedian incision
paraneoplastic syndrome
paranephric abscess
paraperitoneal nephrectomy
paraphimosis
paraprostatitis
parasitic chylocele
paraspadia, paraspadias
parastomal hernia
parasympatholytic drugs
parasympathomimetic drugs
paratesticular
> rhabdomyosarcoma

parauresis

Paredrine
parenchyma
parenchymal
   p. sparing surgery
   p. tumor
parenteral
   p. guanethidine
   p. methyldopa
   p. nutrition
pargyline
Parkinson's disease
Parnate
parorchidium
Parsidol
partial
   p. cystectomy
   p. nephrectomy
partial-occlusion clamp
particulate silicone
paruresis
passive incontinence
Pasteurella
   P. multocida
patch
   p. angioplasty
   aortic p.
   Carrel aortic p.
   p. graft
   vein p.
patency
   p. rate
patent urachus
Pathilon
pathogenesis
pathologic substaging
patient selection
pattern
   echo p.
Pavabid
Pavacap
Pavacen
Pavatest
Pavatine

PCNA
   proliferating cell nuclear
   antigen
PCNL
   percutaneous
   nephrolithotomy
PDS suture
peak response
pediatric carcinoma
pedicle
   renal p.
   vascular p.
pediculicide
pediculosis
pefloxacin
pelvic
   p. brim
   p. exenteration
   p. floor movement
   p. lymphadenectomy
   p. muscle training
   p. stone
pelvicaliceal
   p. stasis
   p. system
pelvilithotomy, pelviolithotomy
pelvioplasty
pelviotomy, pelvitomy
pelvis
   arcus tendineus
     fasciae p.
   obstructed p.
   renal p.
pelviscope
pelvitomy (*var. of*
   pelviotomy)
penbutolol
pencil-tipped electrode
pendiomide
penectomy
Penetrak
penetration
   capsular p.
Penetrex

penicillamine
penile
    p. amputation
    p. carcinoma
    p. duplex
      ultrasonography
    p. erection
    p. extensibility
    p. fibromatosis
    p. implant
    p. incarceration
    p. injection testing
    p. injection therapy
    p. plethysmography
    p. revascularization
    p. torsion
    p. urethra
    p. vascular function
      assessment
    p. vein occlusion
      therapy
    p. venous ligation
      surgery
penile-brachial index
penis
    bifid p.
    clubbed p.
    double p.
    p. lunatus
    p. palmatus
    webbed p.
penischisis
penitis

Penn pouch
penoscrotal
    p. hypospadias
    p. transposition
penotomy
Penrose drain
pentapiperium
pentazocine
penthienate
pentolinium
pentoxifylline
peptichemio (PTC)
peptide
    calcitonin gene
      related p. (CGRP)
    vasoactive intestinal p.
      (VIP)
percutaneous
    p. debulking
    p. drainage
    p. embolization therapy
    p. needle aspiration
    p. nephrolithotomy
      (PCNL)
    p. nephrostomy
    p. stone removal
    p. transcatheter
      perfusion
    p. transluminal
      angioplasty
    p. transluminal renal
      angioplasty (PTRA)
    p. ultrasonic lithotriptor

NOTES

Pereyra
  P. bladder neck
    suspension
  P. ligature carrier
  P. procedure
perforating forceps
perforation
  bladder p.
perfusate
  p. bag
  hyperosmolar p.
  p. solution
perfusion
  continuous hypothermic
    pulsatile p.
  p. cooling
  hypothermic p.
  p. machine
  percutaneous
    transcatheter p.
  transcatheter p.
  transvenous p.
  trickle p.
perimedial fibroplasia
perinea (*pl. of* perineum)
perineal
  p. descent
  p. hypospadias
  p. incision
  p. lithotomy
  p. nerve
  p. prostatectomy
  p. section
  p. urethrostomy
  p. urethrotomy
  p. urinary fistula
perineobulbar
  p. detrusor facilitative
    reflex
  p. detrusor inhibitory
    reflex
**perineodetrusor inhibitory
  reflex**
perineostomy

perineotomy
perinephric
  p. abscess
perineum, pl. perinea
  watering-can p.
perioperative
  p. nutrition
periprostatic
  p. tissue
perirenal
  p. abscess
  p. hematoma
peritomy
peritoneal
  p. dialysis
  p. window
peritoneoscopy
peritoneotomy
  inverted V p.
peritoneum
peritonitis
  meconium p.
periureteral
  p. abscess
  p. fibrosis
periureteritis
  p. plastica
periurethral
  p. abscess
  p. striated muscle
perivesical fat
Permitil
perphenazine
Pertofrane
pervenous pacemaker
pessary
  Smith-Hodge p.
Petersen's bag
Peyronie's disease
Pezzer catheter
Pfannenstiel incision
phallalgia
phallectomy
phallitis

phalloarteriography
phallocampsis
phallocrypsis
phallodynia
phalloplasty
phallorrhagia
phallorrhea
phallotomy
pharmacoangiography
pharmacoarteriography
pharmacocavernosogram
pharmaco-duplex
   ultrasonography
pharmacokinetics
phenacetin
phenazopyridine hydrochloride
phendimetrazine
phenelzine
Phenergan
phenindamine
phenmetrazine
phenobarbital
phenol
phenomenon, pl. phenomena
   cloud p.
   Goldblatt p.
   jet stream p.
phenothiazine
phenotype
phenotypic sex
Phenoxine
phenoxybenzamine
phentermine

phentolamine
   p. test
phenylephrine
phenylethylamine N-methyl
   transferase (PNMT)
phenylpropanolamine
phenylpropylmethylamine
pheochromocytoma
   familial p.
Phillips' catheter
phimosis, pl. phimoses
phimotic
phlebitis
phleborrheograph
   Cranley p.
phleborrheography
phlegmonous abscess
pholedrine
phonorenogram
phosphatase
   placental alkaline p.
   (PIAP)
   prostatic acid p. (PAP)
phosphate
   calcium p.
   estramustine p.
   magnesium
   ammonium p.
phosphorous-31 magnetic
   resonance spectroscopy
photochemotherapy
photodynamic therapy
photometer
   transurethral resection

NOTES

photometer *(continued)*
  TUR-Cue p.
    transurethral resection
photomicrography
photon
photosensitizer
  porphyrin p.
phthiriasis
Phthirus pubis
phytonadione
PIAP
  placental alkaline
    phosphatase
Pick's tubular adenoma
piezoelectric
  p. lithotripsy
  p. lithotriptor
  p. shock wave
    lithotriptor
pigtail nephrostomy tube
pilonidal
  p. cyst
  p. sinus
PIN
  prostatic intraepithelial
    neoplasia
pindolol
pipenzolate
piperidolate
piperoxan
Pipradol
piston-type syringe
pituitary tumor
placebo effect
placement
  five-port "fan" p.
  four-port "diamond" p.
  graft p.
placental alkaline phosphatase
  (PIAP)
plane
  cleavage p.
  p. of dissection
planimetry

planuria
plaque
  atherosclerotic p.
  augmentation p.
  ostial atherosclerotic p.
plasma
  p. albumin
  p. cell balanitis
  cryoprecipitated p.
  p. flow
  p. protein fraction
plasmacytoma
plasmid
plasty
  Foley Y-V p.
  posterior bladder flap p.
  Y-V p.
plate
  cloacal p.
  trigonal p.
plateau response
platinum
platinum-based consolidation
  chemotherapy
platinum, Velban and
  bleomycin (PVB)
Plegine
plethora
plethysmography
  penile p.
plexus
  distal venous p.
  longitudinal subepithelial
    venous p.
  proximal venous p.
  suburothelial nerve p.
plication
  Kelly p.
  Nesbit p.
  p. suture
ploidy analysis
Plus
  Ensure P.
  Lithostar P.

PNET
    primitive neuroectodermal
    tumor
pneumatic
    p. compression device
    p. leg pump
pneumatinuria
pneumaturia
pneumography
    retroperitoneal p.
pneumopenis
pneumoretroperitoneum
pneumoscrotum
PNMT
    phenylethylamine N-methyl
    transferase
pocketed calculus
podofilox
point
    F2 focal p.
pointer
    LaserMed laser p.
POINTER computer program
Poiseuille's law
polarization microscopy
polidocanol
Politano-Leadbetter
    P.-L. anastomosis
    P.-L. tunnel creation
    P.-L. ureterolysis
pollakisuria
pollakiuria
polyamine spermine
polyarteritis nodosa

Polycitra
Polycitra-K
Polycitra-LC
polycystic kidney disease
polycythemia vera
polydioxan
polydioxanone
polydipsia
polyethylene glycol
polyglactin
    p. suture
polyorchism, polyorchidism
polypeptide
    vasoactive intestinal p.
    (VIP)
polypropylene suture
polysaccharide Kreha (PSK)
Polytef
Polytef injection
polytetrafluorethylene
    p. paste injection
polytetrafluoroethylene
polyuria
Pondimin
Poole suction tube
Porges catheter
porotomy
porphyrin photosensitizer
port
    inlet p.
    MCL p.
    subcostal p.
    suprapubic p.
    umbilical p.

NOTES

portable renal preservation
machine
position
    dorsal lithotomy p.
    flank p.
    Scultetus' p.
    semioblique p.
    supine p.
posterior
    p. approach
    p. bladder flap plasty
    p. exenteration
    p. lumbar approach
    p. nephrectomy
    p. pelvic exenteration
    p. transthoracic incision
    p. urethra
    p. urethral valve (PUV)
posthetomy
posthioplasty
posthitis
postholith
postinflammatory contracture
postmicturition
    p. continuous leakage
    p. dribble
post-obstructive diuresis
postoperative
    p. complication
    p. hydrocele
post-prostatectomy incontinence
postureteroscopic manipulation
Pos-T-Vac
    P.-T.-V. vacuum
      erection device
    P.-T.-V. VCD
potassium
    p. citrate
potency
    erectile p.
potential
    evoked p.
Potter facies

Potts
    P. forceps
    P. scissors
pouch
    Benchekroun p.
    Bricker p.
    Denis Browne p.
    Duke p.
    Florida p.
    ileocolonic p.
    Indiana p.
    Kock p.
    Mainz p.
    Mainz p. II
    Miami p.
    Penn p.
    sigma rectum p.
    superficial inguinal p.
    Tena p.
pouchogram
pouchoscopy
powder pyelogram
p_2 penile brachial index
PPTT
    prepubertal testicular tumor
Prader orchidometer
pralidoxime
prazosin
preadventitial dissection
precancerous lesion
Precision-HN
Precision-LR
predisposition
    genetic p.
prednisolone
prednisone
pregnancy
    voluntary interruption
      of p. (VIP)
Preludin
Premarin
premature ejaculation
premicturition pressure

Prempree Modification staging
   system
prenatal diagnosis
preparation
   Nichol's bowel p.
prepubertal testicular tumor
   (PPTT)
prepuce
preputial
   p. calculus
prerectal lithotomy
preservation
   extracorporeal p.
   extracorporeal renal p.
   renal p.
   p. time
   p. times effect
pressure
   abdominal p.
   p. amplitude modulation
   bladder p. (BP)
   blood p. (BP)
   detrusor p.
   intraluminal urethral p.
   intraurethral p.
   intravesical p.
   leak point p.
   premicturition p.
   p. regulated
   electrohydraulic
   lithotripsy
   p. transmission ratio
   (PTR)
   ureteral p.

pressure-flow
presurgical medical evaluation
preventive intravesical therapy
priapism
priapitis
prilocaine
primary
   p. obstructive
   megaureter
   p. renal calculus
   p. transitional cell
   carcinoma
priming
   androgen p.
primitive neuroectodermal
   tumor (PNET)
Primus transrectal
   thermography
principle
   Heineke-Mikulicz p.
   Mitrofanoff p.
printer
   Mavigraph color
   video p.
Priscoline
probe
   CO_2 laser p.
   Corson needle
   electrosurgical p.
   Doppler p.
   electrohydraulic
   lithotriptor p.
   electrosurgical p.

NOTES

probe *(continued)*
  electrosurgical monopolar
    spatula p.
  end-fire transrectal p.
  endorectal p.
  p. gorget
  KTP laser p.
  rectal p.
  transrectal p.
  ultrasonic lithotriptor p.
procaine hydrochloride
procarbazine
procedure *(See also* operation,
  repair)
  Al-Ghorab p.
  antireflux p.
  Boari bladder flap p.
  Camey p.
  Cecil p.
  Chester-Winter p.
  dartos pouch p.
  Datta p.
  Devine-Devine p.
  Ebbehoj p.
  Fowler-Stephens p.
  Gilchrist p.
  Gil-Vernet p.
  Goulding p.
  Gregoir-Lich p.
  Halban p.
  Hinman p.
  Hodgson technique of
    modified Lich p.
  island flap p.
  Johnston p.
  Johnston buttonhole p.
  Leadbetter p.
  Lich p.
  Marshall-Marchetti-
    Krantz p.
  Mathieu p.
  Maydl p.
  Michal I p.
  Michal II p.

  Moschcowitz p.
  Nesbit p.
  one-stage p.
  Pereyra p.
  Raz p.
  Richardson p.
  Spence p.
  Stamey p.
  suburethral sling p.
  Thompson p.
  Winter p.
processing
  image p.
prochlorperazine
proctitis
proctocystocele
proctocystoplasty
proctocystotomy
proctosigmoidoscopy
procyclidine
profile
  resting urethral
    pressure p.
  stress urethral
    pressure p.
  urethral closure
    pressure p.
  urethral pressure p.
progesteronal agent
progesterone
prognosis
prognostic factor
program
  CLIM computer p.
  POINTER computer p.
  Stat-View 512
    computer p.
progressive toxicity
Project
  National Prostatic
    Cancer P.
prolactin
Prolamine

prolapse
   genitourinary p.
   stomal p.
   urethral p.
Prolene suture
Proleukin
   P. aldesleukin
proliferating
   p. cell
   p. cell nuclear antigen
    (PCNA)
proliferation
   cell p.
   diffuse mesangial p.
Prolixin
Proloprim
promazine
promethazine
Promex biopsy needle
propantheline
prophylactic lymphadenectomy
prophylaxis
   antibiotic p.
   antimicrobial p.
propranolol
propylhexedrine
Proscan ultrasound imaging
  system
Proscar
Pros-Check kit
Prosed/DS
prospermia
prostaglandin
   p. E_1

prostaglandin E
Prostakath urethral stent
prostatalgia
prostate
   p. balloon dilator
   transurethral laser
    incision of the p.
    (TULIP)
prostatectomy
   cavernous nerve-
    sparing p.
   nerve-sparing radical p.
   perineal p.
   radical p.
   radical perineal p.
   radical retropubic p.
   Stanford radical
    retropubic p.
   suprapubic p.
   total perineal p.
   transurethral p.
   transurethral ultrasound
    guided laser induced p.
    (TULIP)
prostate-specific
   p.-s. antigen (PSA)
   p.-s. antigen density
    (PSAD)
Prostathermer
   Biodan P.
   P. 99D
Prostathermer prostatic
  hyperthermia system

NOTES

prostatic
  p. acid phosphatase
    (PAP)
  p. adenocarcinoma
  p. adenoma
  p. calculus
  p. capsule
  p. carcinoma
  p. catheter
  p. chips
  p. fossa
  p. hyperplasia
  p. hypertrophy
  p. intraepithelial
    neoplasia (PIN)
  p. massage
  p. neoplasm
  p. stent
  p. urethra
  p. urethral transitional
    cell carcinoma
  p. utricle
  p. volume
prostatism
prostatitic
prostatitis
  chronic p.
  granulomatous p.
  nonbacterial p.
prostatocystitis
prostatocystotomy
prostatodynia
prostatolith
prostatolithotomy
prostatomegaly
prostatomy
prostatorrhea
prostatoseminal vesiculectomy
prostatotomy
prostatovesiculectomy
prostatovesiculitis
prosthesis
  Alpha I inflatable
    penile p.

AMS Hydroflex
  penile p.
AMS 600 malleable
  penile p.
AMS 700 penile p.
AMS Ultrex penile p.
Duraphase penile p.
Dynaflex penile p.
Flexi-Flate II penile p.
Flexi-Flate I penile p.
Flexirod penile p.
G.F.S. Mark II
  inflatable penile p.
Hydroflex penile p.
Jonas penile p.
Mentor-Alpha I
  penile p.
Mentor inflatable
  penile p.
Mentor IPP p.
Omniphase penile p.
Scott penile p.
Small-Carrion penile p.
Ultrex Plus penile p.
Unitary inflatable
  penile p.
Urolume p.
prosthetic
  p. arterial graft
  p. bladder
prosthetics
Protalba-R
protamine
  p. sulfate
protease
  p. inhibitor
protein
  C-reactive p.
  p. metabolism
  Tamm-Horsfall p.
  urinary marker p.
proteinuria
proteoglycans
proteolytic

Proteus
prothrombin time
protocol
    clinical p.
    treatment p.
Protokylol
Protopam
protriptyline
Providencia
proxetil
    cefpodoxime p.
proximal
    p. venous plexus
prune belly syndrome
PS-2 needle
PSA
    prostate-specific antigen
    PSA index
PSAD
    prostate-specific antigen
    density
pseudoaneurysm
    p. formation
pseudocapsule
pseudocryptorchism
pseudodiverticula
pseudoephedrine
pseudohermaphroditism
pseudolymphoma
Pseudomonas
    P. aeruginosa
pseudoneurogenic bladder
PSK
    polysaccharide Kreha

psoas
    p. hitch
    p. muscle
psychogenic impotence
psychological support
psychosexual support
psychotropic drug
psychrophore
PTC
    peptichemio
PTR
    pressure transmission ratio
PTRA
    percutaneous transluminal
    renal angioplasty
pubis
    Phthirus p.
    symphysis p.
pubococcygeal muscle training
pubococcygeus muscle
puboprostatic sling
puborectalis sling
pubourethral ligaments
pubovaginal sling
pucker
pudendal
    p. nerve
    p. nerve terminal motor
    latency
pulmonary embolism
pulsatile hematoma
pulsed Doppler
pulsed-dye neodymium:YAG
    laser

NOTES

pulse volume recording
pulverizer
  Thermovac tissue p.
pump
  AS 800 p.
  Bluemle p.
  calcium ATPase p.
  Harvard p.
  infusion p.
  pneumatic leg p.
  roller p.
punch
  aortic p.
  biopsy p.
puncture
  calix p.
  cystic p.
purine
  dietary p.
purpura
  Henoch-Schoelein p.
pusher
  ENDO-ASSIST reusable
   knot p.
  Gazayerli knot p.
  metal-tipped stent p.
PUV
  posterior urethral valve
PVB
  platinum, Velban and
   bleomycin
pyelectasis, pyelectasia
pyelitic
pyelitis
pyelocaliectasis
pyelocalycotomy
pyelocystitis
pyelofluoroscopy
pyelogram
  antegrade p.
  intravenous p. (IVP)
  powder p.
  retrograde p.

pyelography
  retrograde p.
pyelolithotomy
  coagulum p.
pyelonephritis
  acute p.
  ascending p.
  chronic p.
  xanthogranulomatous p.
pyelonephrosis
pyeloplasty
  Anderson-Hynes p.
  Anderson-Hynes
   dismembered p.
  capsular flap p.
  Culp p.
  Culp spiral flap p.
  disjoined p.,
   dismembered p.
  Foley Y-plasty p.
  Scardino vertical flap p.
  Thompson capsule
   flap p.
pyeloplication
pyeloscopy
pyelostomy
pyelotomy
  extended p.
  open p.
pyeloureteral catheter
pyeloureterectasis
pyeloureterography
pyeloureterostomy
pyelovenous
pyelovesicostomy
pyloric stenosis
pyocystis
pyocystitis
pyonephritis
pyonephrolithiasis
pyonephrosis
pyopyelectasis
pyosemia
pyospermia

pyoureter
Pyraminyl
pyrexia
Pyribenzamine
pyridostigmine
pyrilamine

pyrimidine
pyrimidinone
Pyrinyl
pyrogen
    endogenous p.
pyuria

NOTES

QAD-1
  Doppler Q.
Q-switched alexandrite laser
Q-tip test

quality of life
Quarzan
quinolone

R-837
racephedrine
radial jaw bladder biopsy
  forceps
radiation
    r. enteritis
    r. therapy
radical
    r. cystectomy
    r. en bloc removal
    r. inguinal orchiectomy
    r. nephrectomy
    r. nephroureterectomy
    r. perineal prostatectomy
    r. prostatectomy
    r. retropubic
      prostatectomy
    superoxide r.
radioactive
    r. cholesterol
    r. seed implantation
radiobiology
radiocolloid
radioenzymatic assay
radiographic triad
radiography
    kidney, ureter,
      bladder r. (KUB
      radiography)
    KUB r.
      kidney, ureter, bladder
      radiography
radioimmunoassay
    Yang PSA r.
radioimmunodetection
radioiodination
radioisotope
    r. renography
    r. scan
    r. scanning
radiolucent
radionecrosis

radionuclide
    r. imaging
    r. renal imaging
radiotherapy
radium-226
ramification
Ramirez Silastic cannula
Randall stone forceps
range
    metabolic r.
    optimum cooling r.
Ransley-Cantwell repair
Rapoport test
rate
    allograft survival r.
    flow r.
    glomerular filtration r.
      (GFR)
    metabolic r.
    mortality r.
    patency r.
    stone-free r.
    survival r.
    voiding flow r.
ratio
    pressure transmission r.
      (PTR)
    renal vein renin r.
Raudixin
Rautina
Rauval
Rauverat
rauwolfia
Rauzide
Raz
    R. bladder neck
      suspension
    R. 4-corner vaginal wall
      sling
    R. modification
    R. procedure

RCU
recurrent calcium
urolithiasis
reaction
Feulgen r.
foreign body r.
**real-time 3-D biplanar
transperineal prostate
implantation**
reanastomosis
end-to-end branch r.
recanalization
receptor
androgen r.
Recklinghausen's tumor
reconstruction
3-D computer r.
recording
pulse volume r.
rectal
r. carcinoma
r. examination
r. fascia
r. laceration
r. probe
r. probe
electroejaculation
rectourethral
r. fistula
r. muscle
rectovesical fistula
rectum irrigation
recurrent
r. calcium urolithiasis
(RCU)
r. focal sclerosing
glomerulonephritis
Rediwash skin cleanser
red rubber catheter
reflex
Babinski r.
brain stem-sacral loop
bulbocavernosus r.

bulbocavernosus r.
(BCR)
detrusodetrusor
facilitative r.
detrusosphincteric
inhibitory r.
detrusourethral
inhibitory r.
r. incontinence
r. neurogenic bladder
r. neuropathic bladder
perineobulbar detrusor
facilitative r.
perineobulbar detrusor
inhibitory r.
perineodetrusor
inhibitory r.
renal r.
skin-CNS-bladder r.
sympathetic sphincter
constrictor r.
urethrodetrusor
facilitative r.
urethrosphincteric
guarding r.
urethrosphincteric
inhibitory r.
reflux
nondilating r.
ureterorenal r.
vesicoileal r.
vesicoureteral r.
registration
transcutaneous r.
Regitine
regression
spontaneous r.
Regroton
regulation
growth r.
rehabilitation
sexual r.
reimplantation
aortorenal r.

Cohen cross-trigonal r.
end-to-side r.
ureteral r.
rejection
acute vascular r.
vascular r.
relaxation technique
release
stimulated r.
remission
remnants
müllerian r.
removal
percutaneous stone r.
radical en bloc r.
Renacidin
R. irrigation
renal
r. abscess
r. adenocarcinoma
r. agenesis
r. allograft
r. arterial occlusive disease
r. arteriography
r. artery aneurysm
r. autotransplantation
r. biopsy
r. calculus
r. capsulotomy
r. carbuncle
r. carcinoma
r. carcinosarcoma
r. cell carcinoma

r. colic
r. cortical adenoma
r. corticoadrenal
r. cyst
r. cyst decortication
r. cystic disease
r. duplication
r. duplication with segmental renal dysplasia
r. epistaxis
r. failure
r. fascia
r. function
r. hematoma
r. hematuria
r. hemophilia
r. hemorrhage
r. hypertension
r. hypothermia
r. injury repair
r. mass
r. pedicle
r. pelvic carcinoma
r. pelvic transitional cell carcinoma
r. pelvis
r. preservation
r. preservation perfusion system
r. reflex
r. revascularization
r. scan

NOTES

renal *(continued)*
  r. thromboendar-erectomy
  r. transplant
  r. transplantation
  r. trauma
  r. tubular acidosis
  r. vascular injury
  r. vein renin ratio
  r. vein thrombosis
Renese
renewal
  tissue r.
renin
renogastric fistula
Renografin
renogram
renography
  captopril r.
  diethylene-
    triaminepentaacetic
    acid r. (DTPA
    renography)
  DTPA r.
    diethylene-
      triaminepentaacetic
      acid renography
  isotope r.
  radioisotope r.
renomegaly
renopathy
renoprival
renorrhaphy
renovascular
  r. hypertension
Renovist
Renovue
reoperative
  ureteroneocystostomy
reoxygenation
repair *(See also* operation,
  procedure)
  Boari ureteral flap r.
  Cantwell epispadias r.

Devine hypospadias r.
  extracorporeal r.
  first-stage r.
  one-stage r.
  Ransley-Cantwell r.
  renal injury r.
  two-stage r.
  vascular laceration r.
reperfusion
  r. injury
replacement
  bladder r.
  intestinal ureter r.
  intestinal ureteral r.
reproduction
  assisted r.
reproductive system
rescinnamine
resection
  bowel r.
  electrocautery r.
  transurethral r.
    (photometer, TUR,
    TUR-Cue photometer,
    TUR-Cue photometer)
  transurethral r. of
    prostate (TURP)
  transverse r.
  wedge r.
resectoscope
  Foroblique r.
  Iglesias r.
  Iglesias fiberoptic r.
  r. loop
  Olympus continuous
    flow r.
  r. sheath
  Wolf r.
resectoscopy
Resercen
reserpine
reservoir
  ileal r.
  ileocecal r.

ileocecal continent
  urinary r.
Indiana continent r.
**Resident Assessment Protocol
for incontinence**
residual
  r. fragment
  r. urine
  r. urine volume (RUV)
resistance
  drug r.
  urethral r.
respiratory burst
response
  peak r.
  plateau r.
rest
  adrenal r.
  ectopic adrenal r.
  Krause arm r.
  testicular adrenal r.
**resting urethral pressure
profile**
retained testis
retention suture
retinoblastoma
retinoid
retractile testis
retractor
  Army-Navy r.
  Balfour r.
  Bookwalter r.
  Bookwalter ring r.
  Crile angle r.

Deaver r.
fan r.
fan-type laparoscopic r.
Finochietto r.
fixed ring r.
Forder r.
Gil-Vernet r.
Greishaber self-
  retaining r.
Harrington Deaver r.
malleable r.
McBurney r.
metal bar r.
Millin bladder r.
ribbon r.
Richardson r.
Scott r.
self-retaining ring r.
vein r.
Wexler r.
Young prostatic r.
retransplantation
retreatment
  lithotripsy r.
retrocecalis tumor thrombus
retrograde
  r. balloon rupture
  r. intrarenal surgery
  r. occlusion balloon
  catheter
  r. pyelogram
  r. pyelography
  r. ureteropyelogram
  r. urography

NOTES

retrohepatic
retroperitoneal
  r. approach
  r. fibrosis
  r. lymphadenectomy
  r. neoplasm
  r. pneumography
  r. tumor
retroperitoneoscopy
retroperitoneum
retroperitonitis
  idiopathic fibrous r.
retropubic urethroscopy
Retzius
  space of R.
reusable laparoscopic electrode
revascularization
  myocardial r.
  penile r.
  renal r.
reversal
rhabdoid tumor
rhabdomyolysis
rhabdomyoma
rhabdomyosarcoma (RMS)
  paratesticular r.
rhabdosphincter
  electromyography
rheumatism
rhizotomy
ribbon retractor
rib cutter
Richardson
  R. procedure
  R. retractor
rifampicin
rifampin
rifamycin
right-angle
  r.-a. clamp
  r.-a. electrode
right-angled end-to-side
  anastomosis

right ovarian vein syndrome
rigid
  r. nephroscope
  r. ureteroscope
rigidity
RigiScan
  R. device
  R. measurement
ring
  Smith r.
Ringer's lactate
"ring-type" rigidity measuring
  device
risk
Ritalin
RMS
  rhabdomyosarcoma
Robertson TM urethroscope
Robinson catheter
Robinul
Rocephin
rod
  ileostomy r.
rod-lens system
roentgenography
roller pump
rormothermic effect
rosebud stoma
Roth Grip-Tip suture guide
routine neonatal circumcision
Rovsing operation
Rumel tourniquet
running suture
rupture
  retrograde balloon r.
Rüsch stent
RUV
  residual urine volume
R wave coordination
Ryle tube

sac
   yolk s.
saccular
   s. aneurysm
saccule
Sach's solution
Sachs urethrotome
sack
   entrapment s.
sacrococcygeal teratoma
sacrotuberous ligament
s-adenosylmethione (SAM)
Safe and Dry panty and pad
   system
safety wire
sagittal image
saline
   s. cystometry
   heparinized s.
   indigo-carmine-stained
      normal s.
   s. slush
salt-losing nephritis
Salutensin
salvage
   s. cystectomy
SAM
   s-adenosylmethione
sand
   urinary s.
Sani Pads medicated
   cleansing pads
Sanorex
Sansert
saphenous
saprophyticus
   Staphylococcus s.
sarcoma
   botryoid s.
   clear cell s.
   Ewing's s.

Kaposi's s.
   osteogenic s.
Satinsky clamp
SBPN
   simultaneous bilateral
   percutaneous
   nephrolithotomy
Scale
   Kaplan-Anderson Quality
      of Well-Being S.
scale
   Charrière s.
   ECOG performance
      status s.
   Karnofsky s.
   Karnofsky performance
      status s.
scalpel
scan
   bone s.
   gallium s.
   isotropic s.
   99mTc-DMSA s.
   99m technetium
      diethylenetriamine
      pentaacetic acid s.
   nuclear isotope s.
   radioisotope s.
   renal s.
   ^{99m}Tc MDP nuclear
      isotope bone s.
   transabdominal s.
   transrectal s.
   transvesical s.
   UJ13A nuclear isotope
      bone s.
Scanner
   Kretz Combison
      Ultrasound S.
scanner
   Bruel & Kjaer s.

scanning
    captopril-DTPA s.
    s. electron microscopy
      (SEM)
    iodine hippurate s.
    radioisotope s.
    transrectal ultrasound s.
      (TRUS)
Scardino
    S. flap
    S. vertical flap
      pyeloplasty
Scarpa's fascia
scarring
    local s.
scavenger
    free radical s.
Schiff stain
Schistosoma haematobium
schistosomiasis
schwannian spindle cell
sciatica
scintigraph
scintigraphy
    dimercaptosuccinic
      acid s. (DMSA
      scintigraphy)
    DMSA s.
      dimercaptosuccinic
        acid scintigraphy
scissors
    cold s.
    dissection s.
    electrosurgical s.
    electrosurgical curved s.
    endoscopic s.
    hook s.
    insulated curved s.
    insulated straight s.
    Mayo s.
    meatotomy s.
    Metzenbaum s.
    Potts s.
    Strulle s.

    suture s.
    Westcott s.
sclerosing solution
sclerotherapy
scoliosis
scopolamine
score
    Gleason s.
    hostility s.
Scott
    S. penile prosthesis
    S. retractor
screening
    cancer s.
    s. cystometry
    endocrine s.
scrota (*pl. of* scrotum)
scrotal hernia
scrotectomy
scrotitis
scrotocele
scrotoplasty
scrotum, pl. scrota, scrotums
    acute s.
    lymph s.
    watering-can s.
Scultetus' position
searcher
secondary
    s. incontinence
    s. metastatic carcinoma
    s. renal calculus
    s. surgery
section
    frozen s.
    perineal s.
Sectral
seeding
    tumor s.
segment
    Ask-Upmark renal s.
    ileocecal s.
segmental renal dysplasia
Segura basket

Seldinger technique
selection
    patient s.
selective targeting
self-catheterization
self-esteem
self-expanding
    s.-e. coil stent
    s.-e. metallic stent
self-image
self-injection therapy
self-monitoring
    nocturnal tumescence s.-m.
self-retaining
    s.-r. catheter
    s.-r. coil stent
    s.-r. ring retractor
SEM
    scanning electron
    microscopy
semen
semiellipsoid
seminoma
    testicular s.
semioblique position
semirigid
    s. endoscope
    s. fiber optic
    ureteroscope
Semken tissue forceps
senna
sensor
    bladder pressure s.

sensory urgency
sepsis
septicemia
Septisol
Septra
septum
    urethrovaginal s.
sequence
    FLASH pulse s.
sequencing analysis
Serentil
series
    Gastrografin GI s.
seromuscular Lembert suture
serotonin
Serpasil
Serpasil-Esidrix
Serratia marcescens
Sertina
Sertoli cell tumor
serum nephritis
set
    dilating s.
    French introducer s.
    introducer s.
    urology s.
sex
    s. hormone binding
    globulin (SHBG)
    phenotypic s.
sexual
    s. differentiation
    s. evaluation

NOTES

① sextant biopsy

sexual *(continued)*
   s. function
   s. rehabilitation
sexually transmitted disease (STD)
Seyd-Neblett perineal template
SGP-2
shadow
   obliteration of psoas s.
sharp dissection
sharp-edged orifice
SHBG
   sex hormone binding globulin
sheath
   Amplatz s.
   nephroscope s.
   resectoscope s.
   ureteroscope s.
   Waldeyer s.
   working s.
shedding
   virus s.
shield
   Active Living incontinence s.
shock
   hypovolemic s.
   s. number
   s. wave
   s. wave lithotripsy
   s. wave lithotriptor
   s. wave treatment
Shohl's solution
shot
   flat low-angle s. (FLASH)
shunt
   Al-Ghorab modification s.
   arteriovenous s.
   cavernospongiosum s.
   cerebral fluid s.
   Hashmat s.

   Hashmat-Waterhouse s.
   s. tubing
   ventriculoperitoneal s.
   vesicoamniotic s.
   Winter s.
side-to-side anastomosis
Siemens
   S. Lithostar
   S. lithotriptor
   S. Somatom DRH CT analyzer
   S. Sonoline ultrasonography
sigma rectum pouch
sigmoid
   s. colon carcinoma
   s. diverticulitis
   s. enterocystoplasty
sigmoidocystoplasty
sigmoidoscopy
sign
   Guyon's s.
Silastic
   S. indwelling ureteral stent
Silber technique
silent thrombosis
silicone
   particulate s.
Silitek Uropass stent
silk
   s. ligature
   s. suture
silver clip
Simplastic catheter
simultaneous
   s. bilateral extracorporeal shock wave
   s. bilateral percutaneous nephrolithotomy (SBPN)
   s. urethral cystometry
Sinequan

single strand conformation
  polymorphism analysis
Singoserp
sinogram
sinus
    pilonidal s.
    urogenital s.
site
    entry s.
    stoma s.
site-specificity
situ
    carcinoma in s. (CIS)
    in s.
Skelaxin
Skene's duct
skin
    s. graft neovagina
    s. tube
skin-CNS-bladder reflex
SL20
    Storz Modulith S.
sleep apnea syndrome
sleeve
    ileal s.
sleeve-type circumcision
sliding
sling
    puboprostatic s.
    pubovaginal s.
    Raz 4-corner vaginal
      wall s.
slit
    dorsal s.

slush
    ice s.
    saline s.
Small-Carrion penile
  prosthesis
smegma
"smiley face" knotting
  technique
Smith-Boyce operation
Smith-Hodge pessary
Smith ring
smoking
    cigarette s.
sodium
    brequinar s.
    ceftriaxone s.
    dantrolene s.
    diclofenac s.
    docusate s.
    estramustine
      phosphate s.
    oxychlorosene s.
soft ice
software
    CODAS s.
    Cytologic s.
    Medtrax Urology s.
    t-EASE s.
solder
    laser tissue welding s.
solid tumor
solitary kidney
solution
    Collins s.

NOTES

solution *(continued)*
  Collins indigo
    carmine s.
  Collins intracellular
    electrolyte s.
  electrolyte flush s.
  GoLYTELY s.
  Krebs' s.
  lavage s.
  normal saline s.
  perfusate s.
  Sach's s.
  sclerosing s.
  Shohl's s.
solvent
somatostatin
sonoelasticity imaging
sonogram
  transverse s.
sonography
  3-D s.
  endoureteral
    ultrasound s.
  high frequency s.
  transrectal s.
Sonoline SI-200/250
  ultrasound imaging system
sonotrode
  s. channel
Sonotrode lithotriptor
soterenol
sound
  Béniqué's s.
  Campbell s.
  Davis interlocking s.
  Greenwald s.
  Jewett s.
  Le Fort s.
  McCrea s.
  Van Buren s.
  Walther s.
Southern blot hybridization
space of Retzius
Sparine

sparteine
spatula
  electrosurgical s.
  s. tip laparoscopic
    electrode
spatulation
  graft s.
specific gravity
specificity
Spectramed transducer
spectrophotometric analysis
spectroscopy
  infrared s.
  magnetic resonance s.
  phosphorous-31 magnetic
    resonance s.
Spence procedure
Spenco padding
sperm
  s. aspiration
  s. yield
spermatic
  s. cord
  s. cord torsion
  s. fistula
spermatocele
spermatocyst
spermatogonia
spermatorrhea
spermine
  polyamine s.
spermolith
sphincter
  AMS 742 artificial
    urinary s.
  AMS 761 artificial
    urinary s.
  AMS 791 artificial
    urinary s.
  AMS 792 artificial
    urinary s.
  AMS 800 artificial
    urinary s.
  artificial s.

artificial urinary s.
double cuff AMS 800
urinary s.
striated s.
sphincterotome
sphincterotomy
transurethral s.
urethral s.
spicule
bony s.
spillage
fecal s.
spinal cord compression
spiral
intraprostatic s.
s. tip catheter
spironolactone
splanchnic
splenectomy
splenorenal
s. bypass
split
s. renal function test
s. thickness skin graft
sponge
absorbable gelatin s.
s. stick
spongiosa
spongiosi
tunica albuginea
corporis s.
spongiositis

spontaneous
s. dissection
s. regression
spoon
s. forceps
s. tip laparoscopic
electrode
spray
DDAVP nasal s.
spreader
meatal s.
squamous cell carcinoma
stage
s. B carcinoma
s. C carcinoma
stages
multiple s.
staghorn calculus
staging
Boden and Gibb
tumor s.
neoplasm s.
operative s.
Stanford s.
stain
Glaxo s.
Kossa s.
Schiff s.
VanGieson s.
staining
Feulgen s.
Stamey
S. colosuspension
S. procedure

NOTES

SPARC procedure - sling for stress urinary incont. in women,

Stamey *(continued)*
S. test
S. tube
Stamm
S. gastrostomy
S. gastrostomy tube
stammering
s. of the bladder
stand
Mayo s.
Stanford
S. radical retropubic prostatectomy
S. staging
stanolone
Staphylococcus
S. epidermidis
S. saprophyticus
staple
metallic s.
stapler
Autosuture s.
CEEA s.
EEA s.
end-end s.
Endo-GIA s.
GIA s.
stasis
pelvicaliceal s.
state
gradient-recalled acquisition in a steady s. (GRASS)
Statham transducer
static
s. cystogram
s. cytophotometry
s. image DNA cytometry
status
fertility s.
ureteroenteric s.
Stat-View 512 computer program

stay suture
STD
sexually transmitted disease
steatorrhea
steinstrasse
Stelazine
stenosis
atherosclerotic s.
atherosclerotic renal artery s.
ileoureteric s.
pyloric s.
ureteroileal s.
vesicoureteric s.
stent
Angiomed blue s.
Angiomed Puroflex s.
antireflux Double-J s.
ASI prostatic s.
Beamer ejection s.
Black Beauty ureteral s.
Braun s.
coil s.
Cook s.
double-J s.
double-J Surgitek catheter s.
double-J ureteral s.
Fader Tip ureteral s.
French double-J ureteral s.
Gianturco metal urethral s.
helical-ridged ureteral s.
Heyer-Schulte s.
intraprostatic s.
J-Maxx s.
Lubri-flex ureteral s.
Microvasive s.
Palmaz s.
Palmaz balloon-expandable s.
Prostakath urethral s.
prostatic s.

Rüsch s.
self-expanding coil s.
self-expanding metallic s.
self-retaining coil s.
Silastic indwelling
  ureteral s.
Silitek Uropass s.
Surgitek s.
Surgitek Tractfinder
  ureteral s.
Surgitek Uropass s.
titanium urethral s.
Universal s.
Urolume prostate s.
Urosoft s.
Urospiral urethral s.
wall s.
Wallstent s.
stenting
  s. catheter
  ureteral s.
stentography
stepladder incision technique
sterile
sterility
  aspermatogenic s.
  dysspermatogenic s.
  normospermatogenic s.
sterilization
sterilize
sternotomy
steroid
stick
  sponge s.

Stilphostrol
stimulated release
stimulation
  s. fork
  transcutaneous electrical
    nerve s. (TENS)
stimulator
  URYS 800 nerve s.
stitch
  baseball s.
  Connell s.
  tagging s.
stochastic knotting
stoma, pl. **stomas, stomata**
  end s.
  loop s.
  Mitrofanoff s.
  rosebud s.
  s. site
stomal prolapse
stone
  s. basket
  bladder s.
  s. burden
  complex s.
  cystine s.
  s. disease
  s. forceps
  s. fragmentation
  hyperoxaluric s.
  impacted s.
  s. impactor
  pelvic s.
  struvite s.

NOTES

stone *(continued)*
  s. surgery
  ureteral s.
stone-free rate
StoneRisk diagnostic test
StoneTrack
storage
  cold s.
  hypothermic s.
Storz
  S. cystoscope
  S. Modulith SL20
  S. nephroscope
  S. syringe
straight
  s. Maryland forceps
  s. mosquito clamp
strangury
strength
  tensile s.
streptokinase
streptozotocin
stress
  s. incontinence
  surgical s.
  s. urethral pressure
  profile
  s. urinary incontinence
striated sphincter
stricture
  bulbomembranous s.
  Hunner s.
  intestinal s.
  ureteral s.
  ureterocolic s.
  ureteroileal s.
  urethral s.
string method for treatment of penile incarceration
strip
  Bio-Gen urine test s.
Strulle scissors
strut
  Mersilene s.

struvite
  s. calculus
  s. stone
STS lithotripsy system
Studer reservoir urinary diversion
Study
  Intergroup
  Rhabdomyosarcoma S.
  (IRS)
  National Wilms'
  Tumor S. (NWTS-4)
study
  bead chain s.
  bulb tip retrograde s.
  flow cytometric s.
  hematologic s.
  molecular s.
  urodynamic flow s.
  voiding s.
stuttering
  urinary s.
  s. urination
subcostal
  s. flank incision
  s. port
  s. transperitoneal
  incision
submucosal
  s. Teflon injection
  s. vaginal muscle
  s. vaginal smooth
  musculofascial layer
substaging
  pathologic s.
substance abuse
substance P
substance S
substitution
  bladder s.
subsymphyseal epispadias
subtraction angiography
subtrigonal
suburethral sling procedure

suburothelial nerve plexus
succinylcholine
sucker
sucralfate
suction
   s. drain
   s. tube
Sudafed
sulcus
   coronal s.
sulfamethoxazole
   trimethoprim and s.
   (TMP/SMX)
sulfate
   dehydroepiandroster-
   one s. (DHAS)
   hyoscyamine s.
   protamine s.
sulfonamide
sulfoxide
   dimethyl s.
sulmarin
Super-Bright microsphere
superficial
   s. inguinal pouch
   s. trigonal muscle
   s. tumor
superinfection
superior mesenterorenal bypass
  technique
superoxide
   s. dismutase
   s. radical
supine position

support
   bladder s.
   emotional s.
   psychological s.
   psychosexual s.
suppression
   immune s.
suppurative nephritis
supraceliac
supradiaphragmatic
supraglottic squamous cell
  carcinoma
suprahilar disease
supralevator
   s. exenteration
suprapubic
   s. cystotomy
   s. cystotomy tract
   urethral atresia
   s. lithotomy
   s. port
   s. prostatectomy
suprarenalectomy
suprarenal Greenfield filter
supravesical urinary diversion
suramin
Suretys
   S. incontinence briefs
   S. pants
   S. panty system
surface cooling
surgeon's knot
surgery
   dialysis access s.

NOTES

Supramontane

surgery *(continued)*
    extracorporeal s.
    intestinal s.
    laser s.
    nephron-sparing s.
    parenchymal sparing s.
    penile venous ligation s.
    retrograde intrarenal s.
    secondary s.
    stone s.
    transsexual s.
    urologic s.
    vascular s.
surgical
    s. drape
    s. flap
    s. incision
    s. loupe
    s. stress
Surgilube lubricant
Surgitek
    S. catheter
    S. Flexi-Flate II penile
      implant
    S. graduated cystoscope
    S. stent
    S. Tractfinder ureteral
      stent
    S. Uropass stent
survival rate
suspension
    bladder neck s.
    Pereyra bladder neck s.
    Raz bladder neck s.
    urethral s.
suspensory bandage
Sustacal
suture
    absorbable s.
    anchoring s.
    chromic s.
    corner s.
    Dexon s.
    s. fatigue

    figure-of-eight s.
    s. guide
    interrupted s.
    Kessler-Kleinert s.
    Lembert s.
    Lembert inverting
      seromuscular s.
    s. ligature
    s. material
    mattress s.
    Mersilene s.
    Monocryl s.
    monofilament s.
    over-and-over s.
    PDS s.
    plication s.
    polyglactin s.
    polypropylene s.
    Prolene s.
    retention s.
    running s.
    s. scissors
    seromuscular Lembert s.
    silk s.
    stay s.
    Teflon-coated Dacron s.
    Tom Jones s.
    traction s.
    vascular s.
swan-neck deformity
swelling
    cell s.
Swiss Lithoclast
sympathetic sphincter
   constrictor reflex
symphysis pubis
symptom
    s. control
    s. index
    irritative s.
    target s.
symptomatic varicocele
Syms tractor
synchondroseotomy

syndrome
abdominal muscle
deficiency s.
acquired
immunodeficiency s.
(AIDS)
Addison s.
adrenogenital s.
Alport's s.
autoimmune
deficiency s.
Beckwith-Wiedemann s.
Budd-Chiari s.
Burnett's s.
cauda equina s.
caudal regression s.
Conn s.
Cushing s.
dialysis disequilibrium s.
dialysis
encephalopathy s.
Down s.
Fraley s.
frequency-urgency-pain s.
Gorlin basal cell
nevus s.
hemolytic uremic s.
hepatorenal s.,
hepatonephoric s.
Hinman s.
Horner s.
Kallman s.
Mayer-Rokitansky s.
megacystic s.

megacystis-megaureter s.
milk-alkali s.
mind-bladder s.
minimal-change
nephrotic s.
multiple endocrine
neoplasia s. (MENS)
myoclonus-opsoclonus s.
nephritic s.
Ochoa s.
paraneoplastic s.
prune belly s.
right ovarian vein s.
sleep apnea s.
Takayasu's s.
Thorn's s.
triad s.
Turner's s.
urethral s.
urofacial s.
Wolfram s.
Youssef s.
**Synergist vacuum erection
device**
synergy
synthetic vascular graft
syphilis
syringe
Leveen s.
Lewy s.
motor s.
Neisser's s.
piston-type s.
Storz s.

NOTES

syringe *(continued)*
   Toomey s.
   tuberculin s.
   Wolff s.
syrosingopine
syrup
   Calcidrine s.
System
   Endotek-Ultra
    Urodynamics S.
system
   autonomic nervous s.
   Beamer injection
    stent s.
   Boyarsky symptom
    scoring s.
   Bruel & Kjaer 1846
    ultrasound s.
   Cell Analysis s.
   classification s.
   close suction drainage s.
   collection s.
   core-cut s.
   Doppler Quantum color
    flow s.
   drug carrier s.
   ductal s.
   endocrine s.
   ErecAid s.
   ErecAid vacuum s.
   fiberTome s.
   Gleason staging s.
   Grabstald (Memorial)
    staging s.
   hemi-Kock s.
   Impact lithotriptor s.
   IMx PSA s.
   Innova s.

   intensified radiographic
    imaging s. (IRIS)
   intrarenal collecting s.
   Kleinert's Safe and Dry
    panty and pad s.
   Kretz ultrasound s.
   Madsen-Iversen
    scoring s.
   Medstone IRIS s.
   Medstone STS
    lithotripsy s.
   Mycotrim triphasic
    culture s.
   Olympus video urology
    procedure s.
   pelvicaliceal s.
   Prempree Modification
    staging s.
   Proscan ultrasound
    imaging s.
   renal preservation
    perfusion s.
   reproductive s.
   rod-lens s.
   Safe and Dry panty
    and pad s.
   STS lithotripsy s.
   Suretys panty s.
   Uro-jet delivery s.
   Uro-Pak s.
   Urotract x-ray s.
   Urovision ultrasound
    imaging s.
   VET-CO vacuum s.
   wolffian müllerian
    ductal s.
Systral

table
    Gerhardt t.
    Urodiagnost x-ray t.
Tacaryl
tachycardia
TAE
    total abdominal evisceration
tagging stitch
TA instrument
Takayasu's
    T. arteritis
    T. disease
    T. syndrome
takedown
    colostomy t.
TALT
    testicular adrenal-like tissue
Tamm-Horsfall protein
tamoxifen
tamponade
    tract t.
Tandem thin-shaft transureteroscopic balloon dilatation catheter
tantalum-182
Taractan
target
    t. localization
    t. symptom
targeting
    selective t.
TBI
    total body irradiation
^{99m}Tc MDP nuclear isotope bone scan
T connector
tearing through
t-EASE software
technetium
technique
    Belt t.
    bench surgical t.

Campbell t.
capsule flap t.
cup-patch t.
Davis t.
Eisenberger t.
en bloc t.
Gil-Vernet t.
Gittes t.
Goodwin-Scott t.
Graves t.
Jones-Politano t.
Keystone t.
Kock's t.
Leach t.
Lich t.
Lich extravesical t.
Meares-Stamey t.
membrane catheter t.
microtransducer t.
Mitrofanoff t.
Moh's microsurgery t.
relaxation t.
Seldinger t.
Silber t.
"smiley face" knotting t.
superior mesenterorenal
    bypass t.
Thomas t.
Thompson t.
two-layer open t.
Wickham t.
xenon-washout t.
Young t.
teeth
    interdigitating t.
Teflon
Teflon-coated Dacron suture
telangiectasia
telescope
    Hopkins t.
teletherapy
    orthovoltage t.

telopeptide
Temaril
temperature
    core t.
template
    Seyd-Neblett perineal t.
Tena pouch
Tenckhoff catheter
tenesmus
teniposide (VM-26)
Tenormin
TENS
    transcutaneous electrical
    nerve stimulation
tensile strength
tension
tension-free anastomosis
Tenuate
Tepanil
teratoma
    sacrococcygeal t.
    t. testicular cancer
teratospermia
terazosin
terbutaline
terminal hematuria
terodiline
Terumo guidewire
test
    Albarran t.
    Allen's t.
    artificial erection t.
    Bio-Gen urine t. strip
    Biotel home screening t.
    Bonney t.
    Clonidine suppression t.
    Cochran-Mantel-
    Haenszel t.
    cough stress t.
    diabetes home
    screening t.
    differential renal
    function t.

differential ureteral
    catheterization t.
direct
    immunofluorescence t.
    (DIF-test)
Fisher exact t.
glycopyrrolate t.
home screening t.
Howard t.
Mann-Whitney t.
Mantel-Haenszel t.
Marshall-Marchetti t.
McNemar t.
metyrapone
    stimulation t.
one-hour office pad t.
phentolamine t.
Q-tip t.
Rapoport t.
split renal function t.
Stamey t.
StoneRisk diagnostic t.
twelve-hour home pad t.
washout t.
Whitaker t.
Wilcoxon rank sum t.
Yang Pros-Check PSA t.
testalgia
testectomy
testes (pl. of testis)
testicle
    cryptorchid t.
testicular
    t. adrenal-like tissue
    (TALT)
    t. adrenal rest
    t. carcinoma
    t. descent
    t. seminoma
    t. tubular adenoma
testing
    histocompatibility t.

penile injection t.
viability t.
testis, pl. **testes**
abdominal t.
appendix t.
cryptorchid t.
ectopic t.
inverted t.
irritable t.
movable t.
obstructed t.
t. redux
retained t.
retractile t.
tunica albuginea t.
undescended t.
testitis
testopathy
testosterone
t. enanthate
Test-Size orchidometer
tetracycline
tetradecapetide
tetrahydrozoline
tetrapalmitate
maltose t.
tetrodotoxin
TTX t.
Texas style two-piece catheter
thamuria
Thephorin
TheraCys
therapeutic value

therapy
adjuvant drug t.
alpha-interferon t.
anticoagulation t.
antimicrobial t.
autolymphocyte t.
biologic t.
biologic response
modifier t.
cytokine t.
drug t.
endocrine t.
external beam
radiation t.
external vacuum t.
hormonal t.
immunosuppressive t.
interferon t.
intracavernous
injection t.
laser t.
neodymium:YAG laser t.
penile injection t.
penile vein occlusion t.
percutaneous
embolization t.
photodynamic t.
preventive intravesical t.
radiation t.
self-injection t.
thrombolytic t.
ultrasound-guided shock
wave t.

NOTES

thermography
Primus transrectal t.
Thermovac tissue pulverizer
Thiersch tube
**thigh graft arteriovenous
fistula**
thihexinol
Thiola
thiopropazate
thioridazine
Thiotepa
thiotepa
thiothixene
thiphenamil
Thomas technique
Thompson
T. capsule flap
pyeloplasty
T. procedure
T. technique
thoracoabdominal
t. approach
t. extrapleural approach
t. incision
t. intrapleural approach
t. retroperitoneal
lymphadenectomy
Thorazine
Thorn's syndrome
thorotrast
three-quarter circle electrode
thrill
thrive
failure to t.
thrombectomy
thrombin
thrombocytopenia
thromboembolic
thromboendarterectomy
renal t.
Thrombogen
thrombolytic therapy
thrombophlebitis

thrombosis
bilateral renal vein t.
renal vein t.
silent t.
thromboxane
thromboxane A_2
thrombus
mural t.
retrocecalis tumor t.
through
tearing t.
TICE BCG
tidal drainage
TIL
tumor infiltrating
lymphocytes
Timberlake obturator
time
doubling t.
preservation t.
prothrombin t.
timolol
tincture of belladonna
Tindal
tiopronin
tip
filiform t.
vessel t.
tissue
adrenal-like t.
t. approximation
connective t.
t. culture
fibroelastic t.
hilar structure scar t.
t. morcellator
periprostatic t.
t. renewal
testicular adrenal-like t.
(TALT)
tissue-specific gene expression
titanium
t. clip
t. urethral stent

GOT A GOOD WORD FOR THE NEXT EDITION OF

THIS STEDMAN'S WORD BOOK?

Help us keep future editions of this **Stedman's Word Book** fresh and up-to-date with new words and new ideas!

What's going on in your field? Are there new terms being used in this specialty? Are there better, easier ways for organizing the book's content?

Be specific! We want to know how we can make this **Stedman's Word Book** the very best specialty medical word reference possible for you. So go ahead and fill-in the lines below with your best thoughts and recommendations. Attach a separate sheet of paper if you have to—*you* are our most important contributor and we want to know what's on *your* mind!

Thanks!

(PLEASE TYPE OR PRINT CLEARLY)

OK, here's what I think: _____

_____

_____

_____

_____

_____

_____

_____

All done? Great, just detach this card and mail today. No postage necessary, and thanks again!

Name _____ Title _____

Facility _____

Address _____

_____

City _____ State _____ Zip _____-_____

Day Telephone No. ( ) _____

Williams & Wilkins
428 East Preston Street • Baltimore, MD 21202-6564

7960-3 UROLOGY

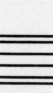

BUSINESS REPLY MAIL

FIRST CLASS   PERMIT NO. 724   BALTIMORE, MD

POSTAGE WILL BE PAID BY ADDRESSEE

Williams & Wilkins
ATTN: REFERENCE DIVISION/Gail Russell
P.O.Box Box 1496
Baltimore, Maryland 21298-9724

TMP/SMX
  trimethoprim and
  sulfamethoxazole
    lomefloxacin TMP/SMX
TNF
  tumor necrosis factor
tocodynamometer
  guard-ring t.
Tocosamine
Tofranil
tolazoline
  t. hydrochloride
Toldt
  white line of T.
Tom Jones suture
tomography
  computed t. (CT)
tongs
tonsil clamp
Toomey syringe
toothed forceps
Toradol
Torek operation
Toronto-Western catheter
torque wire
torsion
  penile t.
  spermatic cord t.
  t. of testis
tortuous
total
  t. abdominal
    evisceration (TAE)
  t. body irradiation (TBI)

  t. cystectomy
  t. hematuria
  t. parenteral nutrition
  t. pelvic exenteration
  t. perineal prostatectomy
  t. prostatoseminal
    vesiculectomy
tourniquet
  t. occlusion
  Rumel t.
towel clip
toxicity
  progressive t.
toxins
  Coley t.
TPH
  transrectal prostatic
    hyperthermia
trabeculation
trachelocystitis
trachomatis
  Chlamydia t.
Tracker catheter
tract
  t. dilation
  genitourinary t.
  t. tamponade
traction
  cephalad t.
  t. suture
tractor
  Lowsley t.
  Syms t.
  Young prostatic t.

NOTES

training
    pelvic muscle t.
    pubococcygeal muscle t.
Tral
tramazoline
Trandate
transabdominal scan
transarterial perfusion cooling
transcatheter perfusion
transcutaneous
    t. electrical nerve
      stimulation (TENS)
    t. registration
transducer
    Spectramed t.
    Statham t.
transfer
    gamete intrafallopian t.
      (GIFT)
transferase
    phenylethylamine N-
      methyl t. (PNMT)
transformation
    neoplastic t.
transfusion
    blood t.
    type-specific blood t.
transglutaminase
transitional
    t. cell
    t. cell carcinoma
    t. epithelium
    t. zone
transluminal
transmitter
    nonadrenergic
    noncholinergic
    inhibitory t. (NANC
    inhibitory transmitter)
Transorb-HN
Transorb-STD
transplant
    kidney t.

    t. nephrectomy
    renal t.
transplantation
    bone marrow t.
    kidney t.
    renal t.
transport
    utrate t.
transposition
    penoscrotal t.
transpubic incision
transrectal
    t. probe
    t. prostatic hyperthermia
    (TPH)
    t. scan
    t. sonography
    t. ultrasonography
    (TRUS)
    t. ultrasound scanning
    (TRUS)
transseptal orchiopexy
transsexual
    t. surgery
transsexualism
transureteroureteral
anastomosis
transureteroureterostomy
transurethral
    t. balloon dilation
    t. laser incision of the
    prostate (TULIP)
    t. prostatectomy
    t. resection (photometer,
    TUR, TUR-Cue
    photometer, TUR-Cue
    photometer)
    t. resection of prostate
    (TURP)
    t. sphincterotomy
    t. ultrasound guided
    laser induced
    prostatectomy (TULIP)

t. ureterorenoscopy
(URS)
transvenous perfusion
transverse
  t. incision
  t. resection
  t. semilunar skin
  incision
  t. sonogram
  t. testicular ectopia
transvesical scan
tranylcypromine
Tratner catheter
trauma
  iatrogenic t.
  renal t.
Traumacal
traumatic
  t. grasping forceps
  t. inflammation
  t. lesion
  t. locking grasper
  t. masturbation
  t. orchitis
  t. renal mass
Travasorb-MCT
Travasorb-Renal
trazodone
treatment
  adjuvant t.
  t. failure
  intracavernosal
  injection t.
  intralesional t.

t. morbidity
neoadjuvant
  antiandrogenic t.
t. protocol
shock wave t.
trench nephritis
Trental
Treponema pallidum
triad
  radiographic t.
  t. syndrome
trial
  clinical t.
Triaminicin
triangle
  femoral t.
triangulation
  t. method
  t. stapling method
triazolam
trichomonal balanitis
Trichomonas vaginalis
tricitrate
trickle perfusion
tricyclamol
tridihexethyl
trifluoperazine
triflupromazine
trigonal plate
trigone
  deep t.
trigonitis
trihexyphenidyl
Trilafon

NOTES

trilobar hyperplasia
trilobar hypertrophy
trimeprazine
trimetaphan
trimethidinium
trimethoprim
   t. and sulfamethoxazole
    (TMP/SMX)
triphasic cystometric curve
triphosphate
   adenosine t. (ATP)
trocar
   Campbell t.
   Cook urological t.
   t. cystostomy
   Ethicon t.
tromethamine
   carboprost t.
   ketorolac t.
Tru-Cut
   T.-C. biopsy
   T.-C. biopsy needle
trunk
   lumbosacral t.
TRUS
   transrectal ultrasonography
   transrectal ultrasound
    scanning
Tru-Trax
tryptophan
   t. metabolism
TT-3 needle
TTX tetrodotoxin
tuaminoheptane
tube
   aspiration and
    dissection t.
   chest t.
   cystostomy t.
   Frazier suction t.
   t. graft
   Medena t.
   nephrostomy t.
   nephrotomy t.

pigtail nephrostomy t.
Poole suction t.
Ryle t.
skin t.
Stamey t.
Stamm gastrostomy t.
suction t.
Thiersch t.
Willscher t.
tuberculin syringe
tuberculocele
tuberculosis
tubing
   t. clamp
   shunt t.
tubular
   t. damage
   t. excretory mass
   t. necrosis
tubulointerstitial fibrosis
TULIP
   transurethral laser incision
   of the prostate
   transurethral ultrasound
   guided laser induced
   prostatectomy
tumescence
   nocturnal t.
   nocturnal penile t.
    (NPT)
tumor
   adenomatoid t.
   adnexal t.
   anaplastic t.
   angiomatoid t.
   bilateral renal t.
   bladder t.
   Buschke-Löwenstein t.
   carcinoid t.
   celiac t.
   t. cell marker
   t. encapsulation
   extracapsular t.
   germ cell t.

t. grading
granulosa cell t.
Grawitz' t.
t. infiltrating
  lymphocytes (TIL)
interstitial cell t. of
  testis
Leydig cell t.
t. location
t. marker
mediastinal t.
t. necrosis factor (TNF)
noninvasive t.
nonseminomatous t.
parenchymal t.
pituitary t.
prepubertal testicular t.
  (PPTT)
primitive
  neuroectodermal t.
  (PNET)
Recklinghausen's t.
retroperitoneal t.
rhabdoid t.
t. seeding
Sertoli cell t.
solid t.
superficial t.
t. suppressor gene
ureteral t.
urethral t.
t. vaccine
virilizing t.

Wilms' t.
  yolk sac t.
tumorigenesis
tumorlet
  Wilms' t.
tunable pulsed dye laser
tunica
  t. albuginea
  t. albuginea corporis
    spongiosi
  t. albuginea corporum
    cavernosorum
  t. albuginea ovarii
  t. albuginea testis
  t. vaginalis
  t. vaginalis blanket wrap
tunic cyst
tunnel
  t. creation
  ureteral t.
TUR
  transurethral resection
    video monitored TUR
turbulent flow
TUR-Cue photometer
  transurethral resection
Turnbull end-loop ileostomy
Turner's syndrome
Turner-Warwick inlay
TURP
  transurethral resection of
    prostate
twelve-hour home pad test

NOTES

two-layer
  t.-l. anastomosis
  t.-l. enteroenterostomy
  t.-l. open technique
two-stage repair
tymazoline

type III incontinence
type-specific blood transfusion
typhloureterostomy
tyramine
tyrosine

UJ13A nuclear isotope bone scan
ulcer
    elusive u.
    Fenwick-Hunner u.
    Hunner u.
Ultrafem pants
ultrafiltration hemodialyzer
UltraKlenz skin cleanser
ultrasonic
    u. diagnosis
    u. fragmentation
    u. lithotresis
    u. lithotripsy
    u. lithotriptor probe
Ultrasonic oscillating bur
ultrasonics
ultrasonography
    color Doppler u.
    Doppler u.
    penile duplex u.
    pharmaco-duplex u.
    Siemens Sonoline u.
    transrectal u. (TRUS)
ultrasound
    u. guided laser
    u. wand
ultrasound-guided
    u.-g. biopsy
    u.-g. shock wave therapy
ultraviolet irradiation
Ultrex
    U. cylinder
    U. Plus penile prosthesis
umbilical
    u. artery
    u. port
    u. port grasper
umbrella
    Mobin-Uddin u.

UMCL
    upper midclavicular line
underactivity
    detrusor u.
underwater spark gap
undescended testis
unilateral subcostal incision
uninhibited
    u. neurogenic bladder
    u. overactive bladder
unit
    Diasonics DRF ultrasound u.
    electrosurgical u.
    Hounsfield u.
Unitary inflatable penile prosthesis
Universal stent
unroofing
unsex
UPJ
    ureteropelvic junction
upper
    u. midclavicular line (UMCL)
    u. tract disease
Urabeth Tabs
urachal
    u. abscess
    u. cyst
urachus
    patent u.
Urapine
urealyticum
    Ureaplasma u.
Ureaplasma
    U. urealyticum
***Ureaplasma* urethritis**
urecchysis
Urecholine
uredema
Urelief

uremia
uremic breath
ureter
    ectopic u.
    impassable u.
    u. implantation
ureteral
    u. carcinoma
    u. catheterization
    u. encasement
    u. meatotomy
    u. obstruction
    u. occlusion balloon
      catheter
    u. orifice
    u. pressure
    u. reimplantation
    u. stenting
    u. stone
    u. stricture
    u. tumor
    u. tunnel
ureteralgia
uretercystoscope
ureterectasia
ureterectomy
    distal u.
ureteric bud
ureteritis
ureterocalicostomy
ureterocele
    ectopic u.
ureterocelorraphy
ureterocervical
ureterocolic
    u. fistula
    u. stricture
ureterocolonic anastomosis
ureterocolostomy
ureterocutaneous fistula
ureterocystanastomosis
ureterocystoscope
ureterocystostomy
ureteroendoscopy

ureteroenteric
    u. status
ureteroenterostomy
ureterogram
    bulb-tipped retrograde u.
ureterography
ureterohydronephrosis
ureteroileal
    u. anastomosis
    u. stenosis
    u. stricture
ureteroileoneocystostomy
ureteroileostomy
ureteroileourethral anastalsis
ureterolith
ureterolithiasis
ureterolithotomy
ureterolysis
    combined u.
    extravesical u.
    intravesical u.
    Lich-Gregoir u.
    Pacquin u.
    Politano-Leadbetter u.
Ureteromat
ureteroneocystostomy
    reoperative u.
ureteroneopyelostomy
ureteronephrectomy
ureteropelvic
    u. junction obstruction
    u. obstruction
ureteropelvic junction (UPJ)
ureteroplasty
ureteroproctostomy
ureteropyelitis
ureteropyelogram
    retrograde u.
ureteropyelography
ureteropyeloneostomy
ureteropyelonephritis
ureteropyelonephrostomy
ureteropyeloplasty
ureteropyeloscope

ureteropyeloscopy
flexible u.
ureteropyelostomy
ureteropyosis
ureterorectostomy
ureterorenal reflux
ureterorenoscope
ureterorenoscopy
transurethral u. (URS)
ureterorrhagia
ureterorrhaphy
ureteroscope
MR-6 u.
MR-9 u.
offset lens u.
rigid u.
semirigid fiber optic u.
u. sheath
Wolf u.
working port u.
ureteroscopy
ureterosigmoid
u. anastomosis
ureterosigmoidostomy
ureterostegnosis
ureterostenoma
ureterostenosis
ureterostoma
ureterostomy
cutaneous u.
high loop cutaneous u.
low loop cutaneous u.

ureterotomy
Davis intubated u.
intubated u.
ureterotrigonoenterostomy
ureterotubal anastomosis
ureteroureteral
u. anastomosis
ureteroureterostomy
ureterouterine
ureterovaginal
u. fistula
ureterovesical junction (UVJ)
ureterovesical obstruction
ureterovesicostomy
urethra
anterior u.
AS 800 male
bulbous u.
devastated u.
intrinsic striated muscle
of the u.
penile u.
posterior u.
prostatic u.
urethrae
compressor u.
urethral
u. atresia
u. carcinoma
u. caruncle
u. closure pressure
profile
u. dilation
u. diverticulectomy

NOTES

151

urethral *(continued)*
  u. diverticulum
  u. electrical conductance
  u. hematuria
  u. hypermobility
  u. obstruction
  u. occlusion
  u. pressure measurement
  u. pressure profile
  u. prolapse
  u. resistance
  u. sphincterotomy
  u. stricture
  u. suspension
  u. syndrome
  u. tumor
  u. vein
urethralgia
urethralis
  crista u.
urethrameter
urethrascope
urethratresia
urethrectomy
urethremorrhagia
urethremphraxis
urethreurynter
urethrin
urethrism, urethrismus
urethritis
  acute u.
  hypoestrogenic u.
  mycoplasma u.
  nongonococcal u.
  Ureaplasma u.
urethrobalanoplasty
urethrocavernous fistula
urethrocele
urethrocystitis
urethrocystometrography
urethrocystometry
urethrocystopexy
urethrocystorectometry
urethrocystoscopy

urethrodetrusor facilitative
  reflex
urethrodynia
urethrogram
urethrograph
urethrography
urethrohymenal fusion
urethrometer
urethropexy
  Marshall-Marchetti-
  Krantz u.
urethrophraxis
urethrophyma
urethroplasty
  onlay island flap u.
urethrorectal fistula
urethrorrhagia
urethrorrhaphy
urethrorrhea
urethroscope
  Robertson TM u.
urethroscopic
urethroscopy
  retropubic u.
urethrospasm
urethrosphincteric
  u. guarding reflex
  u. inhibitory reflex
urethrostaxis
urethrostenosis
urethrostomy
  perineal u.
urethrotome
  Otis u.
  Sachs u.
urethrotomy
  external u.
  internal u.
  perineal u.
urethrovaginal
  u. fistula
  u. septum
urethrovesicopexy
Urex

urge incontinence
urgency
   idiopathic sensory u.
   u. incontinence
   motor u.
   sensory u.
uric
   u. acid
   u. acid calculus
   u. acid infarct
   u. acid lithiasis
Uricult
Uridium
Urifon-Forte
Urigen
urinal
   "Millie" female u.
   Uro-Tex McGuire
     male u.
   URSEC u.
urinalysis
urinary
   u. calculus
   u. catheterization
   u. cyst
   u. diversion
   u. excretion
   u. exertional
     incontinence
   u. extraversion
   u. fistula
   u. incontinence
   u. marker protein

   u. sand
   u. stress incontinence
   u. stuttering
   u. tract infection (UTI)
   u. umbilical fistula
urinary diversion
   ileocolonic pouch u. d.
   Le Bag u. d.
urination
   stuttering u.
urine
   u. culture
   residual u.
   u. vanillylmandelic acid
urinoma
Urised
Urisedamine
Urispas
Uritrol
Urizole
Urobak
Urobiotic
Uro-Bond skin adhesive
urocele
urocheras
urochesia
Urocit-K
Urocystin
urocystitis
Urodiagnost x-ray table
urodynamic
   u. dysfunction
   u. flow study

NOTES

urodynamics
  ambulatory u.
urodynia
urodysfunction
uroedema
urofacial syndrome
Uroflometer
  Drake U.
Uroflow index
uroflowmeter
  Dantec Urodyn 1000 u.
uroflowmetry
  home u.
urogenital
  u. diaphragm
  u. fistula
  u. sinus
  u. sphincter muscle
Urogesic
urogram
  intravenous u.
urograph
  DISA 5500 u.
urography
  antegrade u.
  cystoscopic u.
  intravenous u.,
    excretory u.
  retrograde u.
Uro-jet delivery system
Urolab Janus System III
urolith
urolithiasis
  asymptomatic u.
  recurrent calcium u.
    (RCU)
urolithic
urolithology
urologic, urological
  u. surgery
urologist
urology
  u. set

Urolume
  U. prostate stent
  U. prosthesis
  U. Wallstent
Uro-Mag
Uro Max II high-pressure
  ureteral balloon dilatation
  catheter
uronate
  glycosaminoglycans u.
    (GAGUA)
  macromolecular u.
    (MMUA)
uroncus
uronephrosis
Uro-Pak system
uropathogen
uropathy
  chronic obstructive u.
  obstructive u.
uroplania
uropsammus
uroscheocele
uroschesis
urosepsis
uroseptic
Urosoft stent
Urospiral urethral stent
urostomy
Uro-Tex McGuire male urinal
urothelial carcinoma
urothelium
Urotract x-ray system
uroureter
Urovision ultrasound imaging
  system
URS
  transurethral
    ureterorenoscopy
URSEC urinal
URYS 800 nerve stimulator,
  pl. **carcinomas, carcinomata**
u-shaped skin flap

uteroscope
    Circon-ACMI u.
UTI
   urinary tract infection
utrate transport

utricle
    prostatic u.
utriculitis
UVJ
    ureterovesical junction

NOTES

VAB
  Velban, actinomycin-D, and
  bleomycin
VAB-II
  Velban, actinomycin-D,
  bleomycin, and platinum
VAB-VI
  cyclophosphamide, Velban,
  actinomycin-D, bleomycin,
  and platinum
VAC
  vincristine, Adriamycin, and
  cyclophosphamide
vaccine
  BCG v.
  irradiated tumor v.
  tumor v.
vacuum
  v. constriction device
  (VCD)
  v. constriction erection
  v. erection device
  v. tumescence device
**vacuum constriction device
  (VCD)**
vaginal
  v. cone biopsy
  v. construction
  v. fistula cup
  v. lithotomy
  v. vesicostomy
vaginalis
  Gardnerella v.
  Trichomonas v.
  tunica v.
vaginalitis
Valethamate
Valpin
Valsalva maneuver
value
  therapeutic v.

valve
  Benchekroun
  hydraulic v.
  v. of Guerin
  ileal nipple v.
  Mitrofanoff v.
  nipple v.
  posterior urethral v.
  (PUV)
Van
  V. Buren sound
van Buren's disease
VanGieson stain
vanillacetic acid (VLA)
vanillylmandelic acid (VMA)
Vantin
variability
varicocele
  symptomatic v.
varicocelectomy
  laparoscopic v.
  microsurgical inguinal v.
varicole
Varicoscreen
vasa deferentia
vasa deferentia (*pl. of* vas
  deferens)
vascular
  v. anastomosis
  v. clamp
  v. injury
  v. invasion
  v. laceration
  v. laceration repair
  v. lesion
  v. pedicle
  v. rejection
  v. renal mass
  v. surgery
  v. suture

vasculogenic impotence
vas deferens, pl. vasa
  deferentia
vasectomy
    no-scalpel v.
vasitis
vasoactive
    v. drug
    v. intestinal peptide
      (VIP)
    v. intestinal polypeptide
      (VIP)
    v. intestinal polypeptide
      immunoreactivity (VIP-
      IR)
vasocutaneous fistula
vasoepididymostomy
vasoligation
vaso-orchidostomy
vasosection
vasospasm
vasostomy
vasotomy
vasovasostomy
vasovesiculectomy
Vasoxyl
VCD
    vacuum constriction device
    Dacomed Catalyst VCD
    Mentor-Piston VCD
    Mentor Response VCD
    Mentor-Touch VCD
    Mission VED VCD
    Osbon ErecAid VCD
    Pos-T-Vac VCD
VCR
    vincristine
VCUG
    voiding cystourethrogram
vein
    aberrant obturator v.
    cavernous v.
    deep dorsal v.
    external spermatic v.

gubernacular v.
internal pudendal v.
v. patch
v. retractor
urethral v.
Velban
Velban, actinomycin-D, and
  bleomycin (VAB)
Velban, actinomycin-D,
  bleomycin, and platinum
  (VAB-II)
vena
    v. cava
    v. cavography
venacavogram
venereal disease
venereum
    lymphogranuloma v.
      (LGV)
venogenic impotence
venography
venous leak impotence
ventriculoperitoneal shunt
ventrocystorrhaphy
ventrum penis flap
venule
vera
    polycythemia v.
verapamil
Veratrum alkaloids
Veress needle
verruca vulgaris
verruciform xanthoma
verrucous carcinoma
Versed
vertical midline incision
verumontanum
vesical
    v. calculus
    v. compliance
    v. diverticulectomy
    v. diverticulum
    v. exstrophy

v. external sphincter
dyssynergia (VSD)
v. fistula
v. hematuria
v. lithotomy
vesical-sacral-sphincter loop
vesicle hernia
vesicoamniotic shunt
vesicocele
vesicoclysis
vesicocolic fistula
vesicocutaneous fistula
vesicofixation
vesicoileal reflux
vesicointestinal fistula
vesicolithiasis
vesico-ovarian fistula
vesicorectal fistula
vesicorectostomy
vesicosalpingovaginal fistula
vesicosigmoidostomy
vesicosphincteric dyssynergia
vesicostomy
cutaneous v.
vaginal v.
vesicotomy
vesicoureteral
v. reflux
vesicoureteric stenosis
vesicouterine fistula
vesicovaginal
v. fistula
v. Holter
vesicovaginorectal fistula

vesicovaginostomy
vesiculectomy
prostatoseminal v.
total prostatoseminal v.
vesiculitis
vesiculoprostatitis
vesiculotomy
Vesprin
vessel
accessory v.
v. dilator
gastroepiploic blood v.
v. tip
vessels
hypoplastic blind-ending
spermatic v.
VET-CO vacuum system
V-flap meatoplasty
viability testing
videocystourethrography
video monitored TUR
videourodynamic evaluation
videourodynamics
vinblastine
vinblastine, actinomycin-D,
and bleomycin (mini-VAB)
vincristine (VCR)
vincristine, Adriamycin, and
cyclophosphamide (VAC)
violet
gentian v.
VIP
vasoactive intestinal peptide

NOTES

VIP *(continued)*
vasoactive intestinal polypeptide
voluntary interruption of pregnancy
VIP-IR
vasoactive intestinal polypeptide immunoreactivity
Virag operation
virilizing tumor
Virilon
virus
molluscum contagiosum v. (MCV)
v. shedding
visceral
Visken
visualization
visual laser ablation
Vital
vitamin
Vivactil
vividiffusion
vivo
ex v.
in v.
Vivonex
Vivonex-TEN
VLA
vanillacetic acid
VM-26
teniposide
VMA
vanillylmandelic acid
voiding
v. cystogram

v. cystometrography
v. cystometry
v. cystourethrogram (VCUG)
v. diary
dysfunctional v.
v. flow rate
v. study
v. urethral pressure measurements (VUPP)
volume
bladder v.
v. overload
prostatic v.
residual urine v. (RUV)
voluntary interruption of pregnancy (VIP)
vomiting
Von
V. Hippel-Lindau cerebellar hemangioblastomatosis
V. Recklinghausen's neurofibromatosis
von
v. Hippel-Lindau disease
VSD
vesical external sphincter dyssynergia
VTU-1 vacuum erection device
vulgaris
verruca v.
vulvar carcinoma
VUPP
voiding urethral pressure measurements

W

Waldeyer sheath
Wallstent
    W. stent
    Urolume W.
wall stent
Walther
    W. dilator
    W. sound
wand
    ultrasound w.
warfarin
washing
    bladder w.
washout test
water
    w. cystometry
    w. displacing balloon
watering-can
    w.-c. perineum
    w.-c. scrotum
wave
    focused shock w.
    shock w.
    simultaneous bilateral
      extracorporeal shock w.
wax-tipped bougie
webbed penis
Weber-Christian disease
weddellite calculus
wedge resection
Weigert-Meyer law
welding
    laser tissue w.
Westcott scissors
Wexler retractor
Wheelhouse operation
whewellite calculus
whistle-tip catheter
Whitaker
    W. hook
    W. test
white line of Toldt

whole body cooling
Wickham technique
wide-angled loupe
wide elliptical anastomosis
Wilcoxon rank sum test
Willscher
    W. catheter
    W. tube
Wilms'
    W. tumor
    W. tumorlet
Wilpowr
window
    peritoneal w.
winged catheter
Winter
    W. procedure
    W. shunt
wire
    flexible tip guide w.
    Glidewire guide w.
    guide w.
    Hydro Plus coated
     guide w.
    J w.
    Lubriglide-coated
     guide w.
    Lunderquist w.
    safety w.
    torque w.
Wolf
    W. lithotriptor
    W. percutaneous
    universal nephroscope
    W. Piezolith 2300
    lithotripsy device
    W. Piezolith lithotriptor
    W. Piezolith 2300
    lithotriptor
    W. resectoscope
    W. Sonolith lithotriptor
    W. ureteroscope

wolffian
>w. duct
>w. müllerian ductal
>system

Wolff syringe
Wolfram syndrome
working
>w. port ureteroscope
>w. sheath

workstation
>Dornier MFL 5000
>urological w.

wound
>w. healing
>w. infection

wrap
>Kerlix w.
>tunica vaginalis
>blanket w.

Wyamine

xanthine oxidase
xanthogranulomatous
   pyelonephritis
xanthoma
     verruciform x.
xenon-washout technique
xiphoid to pubis midline
   abdominal incision

x-ray
     x.-r. diffractometry
XX male mosaicism
Xylocaine
     X. jelly
xylometazoline
xyphoid

Y

YAG laser
Yang
    Y. polyclonal assay
    Y. Pros-Check PSA tet
    Y. PSA
        radioimmunoassay
Y chromosome
90Y-CYT-356
yield
    sperm y.
Yocon
yohimbine hydrochloride

Yohimex
yolk
    y. sac
    y. sac tumor
Young
    Y. needle holder
    Y. prostatic retractor
    Y. prostatic tractor
    Y. technique
Youssef syndrome
yttrium-90
Y-V plasty

Zeppelin clamp
Zipser penile clamp
Zoladex
zona glomerulosa
zona pellucida

zone
    transitional z.
Zoon's erythroplasia
Z-plasty
Zyderm

Appendix 1
Transurethral Resection of Prostate (TURP)

Adson clamp
Adson forceps
Alexander elevator
Ancef
Betadine
bilobar hyperplasia
bilobar hypertrophy
CBI — continuous bladder
  irrigation
cellules
continuous bladder irrigation (CBI)
diverticula
Ellik evacuator
Foley catheter
Foroblique resectoscope
Marcaine
Maxaquin
Mayo scissors
Metzenbaum scissors
nocturia

oblique obturator
prostate-specific antigen (PSA)
prostatic capsule
prostatic chips
prostatic fossa
prostatic hyperplasia
prostatic hypertrophy
PSA — prostate-specific antigen
resectoscope loop
resectoscope sheath
Septisol
Timberlake obturator
towel clip
trabeculation
trilobar hyperplasia
trilobar hypertrophy
ureteroscope sheath
Van Buren sound
verumontanum

Appendix 2
Cystoscopy

Ancef
anterior urethra
Betadine
bladder outlet obstruction
cellules
diverticula
Marcaine
Maxaquin

median bar formation
posterior urethra
prostatic urethra
Septisol
Storz cystoscope
trigonitis
Walther sound
Xylocaine jelly